Beyond Self-Care for Helping Professionals

Beyond Self-Care for Helping Professionals is an innovative guide to professional self-care focused not just on avoiding the consequences of failing to take care of oneself, but on optimal health and positive psychology. This new volume builds upon the Expressive Therapies Continuum to introduce the Life Enrichment Model, a strengths-based model that encourages mindful participation in a broad array of enriching experiences. By enabling therapists and other Helping Professionals to develop a rich emotional, intellectual, and creative foundation to their lives and clinical practices, this guide sets a new standard for self-care in the helping professions.

Lisa D. Hinz, PhD, ATR-BC, is an adjunct professor of art therapy at Notre Dame de Namur University and the author of many professional publications on art therapy.

Beyond Self-Care for Helping Professionals

The Expressive Therapies Continuum and the Life Enrichment Model

LISA D. HINZ

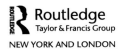

NEW YORK AND LONDON

First published 2019
by Routledge
711 Third Avenue, New York, NY 10017

and by Routledge
2 Park Square, Milton Park, Abingdon, Oxon, OX14 4RN.

Routledge is an imprint of the Taylor & Francis Group, an informa business

© 2019 Taylor & Francis

The right of Lisa D. Hinz to be identified as author of this work has been asserted by her in accordance with sections 77 and 78 of the Copyright, Designs and Patents Act 1988.

All rights reserved. No part of this book may be reprinted or reproduced or utilised in any form or by any electronic, mechanical, or other means, now known or hereafter invented, including photocopying and recording, or in any information storage or retrieval system, without permission in writing from the publishers.

Trademark notice: Product or corporate names may be trademarks or registered trademarks, and are used only for identification and explanation without intent to infringe.

Library of Congress Cataloging-in-Publication Data
Names: Hinz, Lisa D., author.
Title: Beyond self-care for helping professionals : the expressive therapies continuum and the life enrichment model / by Lisa D. Hinz.
Description: New York : Routledge, 2018. |
Includes bibliographical references and index.
Identifiers: LCCN 2018014438 (print) | LCCN 2018034686 (ebook) |
ISBN 9781315316444 (eBook) | ISBN 9781138230996 (hardback) |
ISBN 9781138231016 (pbk.) | ISBN 9781315316444 (ebk)
Subjects: LCSH: Self-care, Health. | Caregivers. | Care of the sick.
Classification: LCC RA776.95 (ebook) |
LCC RA776.95 .H465 2018 (print) | DDC 613—dc23
LC record available at https://lccn.loc.gov/2018014438

ISBN: 978-1-138-23099-6 (hbk)
ISBN: 978-1-138-23101-6 (pbk)
ISBN: 978-1-315-31644-4 (ebk)

Typeset in Dante and Avenir
by Florence Production Ltd, Stoodleigh, Devon, UK

I do not believe that we can put into anyone ideas which are not in him already. As a rule there are in everyone all sorts of good ideas, ready like tinder. But much of this tinder catches fire, or catches it successfully, only when it meets some flame or spark from outside, i.e., from some other person. Often, too, our own light goes out, and is rekindled by some experience we go through with a fellow man. Thus we have each of us cause to think with deep gratitude of those who have lighted the flames within us.

(Schweitzer, 1959, p. 17)

This book is dedicated with love

    to Holly Feen-Calligan who created a spark,

    to George Sakopoulos who protected the flame,

    to Maria Riccardi who fanned the fire,

    to Elena Sakopoulos who carried the torch across the finish line,

    and to Sofia Sakopoulos who starts a fire wherever she goes.

Contents

List of Figures xi
List of Plates xii
About the Author xiii
Preface xv

1 Perils of the Helping Professions — 1
Definitions and Distinctions — 4
Development of Secondary Traumatic Stress and
  Compassion Fatigue — 5
Prevention and Treatment of Secondary Traumatic Stress
  and Compassion Fatigue — 6
Summary and Conclusions — 7
Art Exploration — 8
Questions for Self-Reflection — 8

2 Beyond Self-Care to Life Enrichment — 11
Benefits of Life Enrichment — 11
Definition of Optimal Health — 14
Summary and Conclusions — 15
Suggestions for Art Reflection — 16
Questions for Self-Reflection — 16

3 The Life Enrichment Model — 17
Movement and Sensation — 18

viii Contents

Routine and Emotion		20
Intellect and Symbolism		21
Creativity		21
Intentional Enrichment		22
Dynamic Balance		24
Summary and Conclusions		24
Questions for Self-Reflection		25
4 Life Enrichment through Sensation		**27**
Olfactory Sensation		28
Sharing Aroma		*29*
Visual Sensation		29
Sharing Beauty		*30*
Tactile Sensation		31
Sharing Touch		*31*
Taste Sensation		32
Sharing Flavor		*33*
Auditory Sensation and Silence		33
Sharing Music		*34*
Sensuality and the Brain		35
Maximizing Sensual Pleasure		35
Summary and Conclusions		37
Sensory Actions and Art Reflections		38
Questions for Self-Reflection		38
5 Life Enrichment through Movement		**39**
Benefits of Exercise		40
Increased Positive Emotions		*41*
Improved Cognitive Functioning		*42*
Enhanced Sleep		*42*
Increased Strength		*43*
Decreased Fatigue		*43*
Rhythmic Movement		44
Sharing Movement		45
Summary and Conclusions		46
Movement and Art Reflections		47
Questions for Self-Reflection		47
6 Life Enrichment through Pattern and Routine		**49**
The Comfort of Routines and Patterns		50

Isomorphism	51
Mandala Coloring	52
Lines Can Aid Meditation	52
Sharing Pattern and Perception	54
Representational Diversity	54
Setting Boundaries	57
Summary and Conclusions	58
Pattern and Routine Art Reflection	58
Questions for Self-Reflection	59

7 Life Enrichment through Emotion — 61

The Purpose of Emotions	62
Increasing Positive Emotions	63
Sharing Emotion	64
Emotion Regulation	65
Emotions and Decision Making	67
Summary and Conclusions	68
Emotional Expression Art Reflection	69
Questions for Self-Reflection	70

8 Life Enrichment through Intellect — 71

Changing Thoughts	72
Increasing Positive Aspects of the Self-Narrative	72
Increasing Self-Affirmation	73
Developing Self-Compassion	74
Enhancing Meaning	75
Curiosity and Learning at Work	77
Leisure Pastimes	78
Fostering Grit	78
Sharing Learning	79
Summary and Conclusions	79
Intellect and Art Reflection	80
Questions for Self-Reflection	81

9 Life Enrichment through Symbolism — 83

Art	85
Sharing Symbols: Rituals	87
Social and Religious Rituals	88
Family Rituals	88
More Experiences with Symbolism	89

	Reading Myths and Stories	89
	Illustrated Books	90
	Poetry	90
	Synchronicity, Animal Encounters, and Dreams	91
	Summary and Conclusions	92
	Symbolism and Art Reflection	93
	Questions for Self-Reflection	93
10	**Life Enrichment through Creativity**	**95**
	Creativity and Flow	96
	Creativity and Play	97
	Creativity and Psychological Growth	98
	Creativity and Connection	99
	Increasing Creativity	99
	Summary and Conclusions	102
	Creativity and Art Reflection	103
	Questions for Self-Reflection	103
11	**Living Optimally: A Deep Well, Wide Margins, and Firm Boundaries**	**105**
	A Deep Well	106
	Replenishing the Well	107
	Wide Margins	109
	Firm Boundaries	110
	Dynamic Balance	113
	Summary and Conclusions	114
	Art Reflections on an Enriched Life	115
	Questions for Self-Reflection	116
	References	117
	Index	131

Figures

3.1	The Life Enrichment Model (LEM): A Pathway to Optimal Health	18
3.2	Life Enrichment Model Circle Assessment	23
6.1	Zentangle: Lines Aid Meditation	53
6.2	Optical Illusions Can Enhance Representational Diversity	56
11.1	Diagram of Boundaries	111

Plates

1	Sharing the Beauty of Sensation
2 *and* 3	Art as a Vehicle for Movement and Stress Release
4	Mandala Coloring for Stress Reduction
5 *and* 6	Emotion Expressed through Imagery
7 *and* 8	Collage: Evaluating Work-Life Balance
9	Animal Encounter: The Crow That Would Not Be Ignored
10	Collage: What it Takes to Nurture Creativity
11	Collage of Awe and Wonder

About the Author
Lisa D. Hinz, Ph.D., ATR-BC

Lisa D. Hinz, Ph.D., ATR-BC is a licensed clinical psychologist and a registered, board certified art therapist. After completing her doctorate at Louisiana State University, Dr. Hinz earned a postdoctoral certificate in art therapy at the University of Louisville where she was privileged to work with Drs. Kagin and Lusebrink, the originators of the Expressive Therapies Continuum. After teaching for 17 years at Saint Mary-of-the-Woods College, Dr. Hinz is now an adjunct professor of art therapy at Notre Dame de Namur University. She is the author of many professional publications in the field of art therapy including two books, *Drawing from Within: Using Art to Treat Eating Disorders* and *Expressive Therapies Continuum: A Framework for Using Art in Therapy*. She is a consultant to the Residential Lifestyle Medicine program at Adventist Health Napa Valley and she has a private practice in art therapy. Dr. Hinz uses the creative process to allow clients to access their inner wisdom, promote creativity and wellness, and facilitate change.

Preface

Several years ago, I was asked to teach a weekend course on the Expressive Therapies Continuum to art therapy students at Wayne State University. As part of the experience, Dr. Holly Feen-Calligan, the director of the art therapy master's degree program, asked me if I would also present an hour-long public lecture on a topic of my choosing. In response to the request, I challenged myself to find a way to make the theory of the Expressive Therapies Continuum (ETC) engaging for individuals outside of the art therapy community. The ETC is a theory that explains the various ways that people process information during art making through their interactions with different media and materials (see Hinz, 2009 or Lusebrink, 1990; 1991). Art therapists believe that the way people use materials to produce images in art therapy mimics the ways that they think, feel, and act in life; therefore, I was certain I could make the subject relevant for a wider audience.

One portion of my work is spent in a residential lifestyle medicine program, so, I was inspired to blend my interests in lifestyle medicine and the ETC by following up on a statement I heard someone make at a continuing education lecture a few years ago. The lecture was about habit change, and the instructor made the comment that one way to ensure behavior change was to enrich the environment. The presenter revealed that in an enriched environment, a person was more likely to take advantage of the many opportunities available and less likely to behave in the previously prescribed manner. It struck me that the ETC could be a way to conceptualize the construction of an enriched environment. Thus, the public lecture for Wayne State University was created and called "Enrich Your Life, Change

Your Life: Live Optimally," focusing on the relationship between life enrichment and optimal health.

The lecture received a warm reception and has continued to inspire me to research and teach the topic of life enrichment ever since. I ascribe to a positive approach to psychology and art therapy, focusing more on augmenting clients' strengths and creating a positive future than on ameliorating a negative past, and thus application of enrichment to the field of self-care was natural and probably inevitable. This approach naturally lends itself to a focus on highlighting what individuals can do to nurture themselves into change (like leading an enriched life) rather than fixing what is broken.

At the 2016 American Art Therapy Association conference in Baltimore, I conducted an informal survey of students and art therapists who visited my book-signing table. To those people who were not there to purchase a book, I presented a small original piece of art and asked whether in return, they would write down one thing they wanted to make sure was included in a book that I was writing about self-care. Thirty-three people wrote a comment, and I have grouped their responses into the sections that follow.

Self-Care as a Life Priority

Far and away, most people were concerned about how to conceptualize self-care and prioritize it enough to put it on their list of priorities. This was somewhat surprising, as I thought the topic of self-care would be a familiar concept with a basic application in most people's lives. Therefore, this first concern about making self-care a priority seems to be a matter of making a cognitive shift that includes creating awareness of why self-care is an integral part of one's professional practice and then expanding the mental landscape to include additional time and brainpower for an important new concept.

Because defining and implementing self-care is so fundamental to professional identity, I believe that the appropriate time to begin this cognitive change is during graduate school. However, because it will mean different things at different points in time, the topic of self-care should be addressed at more than one time during graduate school education and throughout the course of a lifetime. At the onset of graduate studies, self-care might seem unnecessary or indulgent as the principal focus throughout this time is on learning content. Theories take precedence and other information can be seen as superfluous. In the middle of graduate school education, students are having some of their first meaningful clinical encounters. Learning therapeutic techniques is all-consuming, and the subject of personal self-care might seem like a distraction from building proficiency.

During the last stages of graduate school, there is greater emphasis on the intensity and nuances of practical work, and self-care might be viewed as important for therapist well-being. However, if this information is newly introduced, it might be experienced as more content to master rather than personally relevant material. Thus, I believe that the topic should be built into learning experiences throughout graduate education and all throughout one's professional career. By the time Helping Professionals are engaged in their clinical practice, the question becomes not the conceptual "what is self-care or why is it important?" but a concrete one: "how do I do it?"

Finding Time

The second theme arising from the survey was a practical one: how to make time for this newly prioritized activity. The majority of participants wrote that they were over-scheduled and did not know how they would add one more activity to an already jam-packed day. This book will explore various ways to fit life-enriching activities into the day without causing additional stress or increasing any perceived sense of burden or responsibility. Some suggestions include increasing mindfulness so that attention is devoted to objects, events, and experiences that increase vitality and joy in life. Further, it is necessary to notice and honor the behaviors that are already in place but might not previously have been considered "self-care" activities. These practices add fullness and richness to life, regardless of what they are called. Also, it is important to note that life-enriching activities do not have to take a great deal of time. A significant effect can be gained through a process called "savoring," which involves spending just 30 seconds completely absorbed in an inspiring activity.

Proactively scheduling self-care activities into the day makes them much more likely to occur. Research shows that creating a "to do" list increases the likelihood of task completion by about 30%, but putting an event into the calendar boosts completion rates to almost 75%. Therefore, enriching activities should have a place on the daily agenda to achieve maximum results. In addition, scheduling activities with friends at a regular set time is another way of making sure that they take place. For example, I schedule a monthly art-making group with friends that fits into our busy schedules and enlivens our lives in a meaningful way. Trying to schedule an informal activity often gets postponed until the "right time;" a scheduled activity is reliably in its "right place" on the calendar. An added bonus of creating in community with loved ones is that the positive effects of this enriching activity are amplified.

Self-Care When It Is Most Needed

The third main point that people who participated in the survey wanted to address was how to make sure that self-care remains a priority when life gets tough or time gets tight. Therapists clearly want to maintain a focus on their own needs, but experience difficulties doing so when their clinical work is focused on putting others' needs first. Related to this theme was the issue of how to avoid "self-sabotage" after successful initial efforts to prioritize and make time for self-care activities. One person wrote that she wanted the equivalent of "Kevlar socks for those of us who shoot ourselves in the foot." Self-sabotage usually results from choosing a behavior with a short-term, positive reward but that has unacknowledged long-term consequences. Therefore, perseverance with self-care efforts requires understanding the positive long-term consequences of life enrichment along with making time for diverse, positive short-term self-care activities. Understanding the importance of life enrichment allows a person to value, invest in, and implement long-term solutions to the potential pitfalls of the helping professions.

Having a broad array of activities to draw from is essential for avoiding self-sabotage and bolstering persistence in self-care and life enrichment endeavors. If you define "self-care" too narrowly, framing it around things like creating art, going out to dinner with friends, or online shopping, those few activities will become increasingly ineffective. We habituate to anything that we do repeatedly – including positive things – and thus, they lose their protective power over time. Thus, it is important to widen the definition of self-care to life enrichment so that many different kinds of experiences can be conceptualized and included. In addition, it is also invigorating to modify a familiar activity to add inspiration. A therapist with whom I worked engaged exclusively in watercolor painting as a form of self-care and after some time, painting began to feel more like a drain rather than a boost to her energy. The negative aspects of her work life began to accumulate in a way that felt oppressive, and she was afraid that she was experiencing professional burnout. At my suggestion she became involved with a life-affirming art-based process called SoulCollage™ and discovered a new reservoir of energy, enthusiasm, and hope for her clinical work.

Changing the medium from watercolor to collage provided this therapist a fresh way of looking at herself, and infused her work with new meaning. A new medium permitted this young woman to explore aspects of herself that were related to her work, while simultaneously allowing her to be separate from her work. In addition, it was an activity that was exclusively for her own enjoyment and enlightenment.

I encourage everyone to change the medium that they work with – both literally if you work with art materials and figuratively with other activities – to make them fresh and rewarding again. Changing the medium also can emphasize the importance of individually defining what life enrichment means to you – there is no set way to create a life that is full of vitality and richness. Your methods, mindfully determined and intentionally employed, will be uniquely yours. This book is replete with examples of life-enriching activities; some will be a perfect fit and others will not fit at all. Some may work at one time and may not work later on. The important thing is that you figure out which activities will work in dynamic balance to invigorate your personal life and professional practice.

Finally, determination in the face of difficulty requires support. This support can be in the form of assistance from a higher power. Knowing that you are not the be-all and end-all of the difficulties that you continuously confront is necessary to sustain perseverance. It is helpful to confide doubts and fears through prayer with a higher power, or in discussion with a supervisor, a therapist, a peer consultation group, or good friend. These interactions can add meaning to struggles and challenges and provide us with inspiration for continuation on the journey.

To summarize, engaging in profoundly nurturing self-care activities is founded upon an understanding of the definition of life enrichment and its necessity for health practitioners. Because of the foundational nature of this information, it is important that it is introduced early in professional education and repeated throughout, as the practice will change over the course of one's career. It also involves practical concerns such as scheduling activities, including friends for support, and varying activities to avoid habituation. Finally, life enrichment involves addressing existential crises and spiritual concerns. All of these themes will be explored in greater depth in the following chapters.

Organization of the Book

The first three chapters of this book introduce the foundation upon which the rest of information is based. Chapter 1 explores the perils of the helping professions including the possibility that without good self-care practices in place, Helping Professionals are at risk for developing various harmful syndromes such as professional burnout, vicarious traumatization, compassion fatigue, and secondary traumatic stress. Definitions of these terms are given and distinctions among them are made. The first chapter ends with a discussion of prevention efforts including life enrichment. Chapter 2 expands upon the concept of life enrichment, with a broad definition of the topic and an exploration of the benefits of living an enriched life. The final part of the chapter discusses the connection between living an enriched life and achieving optimal health, which is proposed as the natural and logical outcome of life enrichment. Chapter 3 introduces the Life Enrichment Model (LEM), which is adapted from the Expressive Therapies Continuum to include a vast array of life-enriching experiences. Each level and component of the LEM is described and the dynamic balance between them discussed. The topic of intentional enrichment as the foundation for self-care and optimal health is addressed.

In-depth discussions of the each component of the Life Enrichment Model are presented in Chapters 4 through 10. The chapters address the dynamic balance between the opposite components on each level and how minding this relationship can further life enrichment. Chapter 4 focuses on the sensation component and how life can be enhanced through various experiences involving vision, hearing, taste, touch, and smell. The effects of sensation are fleeting, so strategies for prolonging and amplifying sensual effects are discussed. Chapter 5 explores movement, which is opposite to sensation on the first level of the LEM. The invigorating physical, intellectual, and emotional aspects of movement are expanded upon, and an important distinction between physical activity and physical exercise is made. Recommendations for life enrichment through physical exercise are suggested.

Chapter 6 focuses on developing the comforting and life-enriching effects of patterns and routines in our lives. The chapter also explores the fact that we take on the feeling of our surroundings, and how we can capitalize on this fact if we are mindful of the physical environment around us. In addition, Chapter 6 addresses three other ways that embracing patterns and routines can fortify our lives: through mandala coloring and other art activities, by developing relational diversity, and through setting and maintaining firm boundaries.

The topic of Chapter 7 is emotion and its purpose in our lives. The chapter includes a discussion of how life enrichment involves both increasing positive emotions and befriending and/or embracing the darker emotions. The importance of communicating emotions is emphasized as the work of positive relationships. Finally, Chapter 7 addresses the topic of emotion regulation and vitalization through art making.

Chapter 8 discusses the difference between left- and right-hemisphere brain functioning then focuses on left-brain functions, called intellect, in the LEM. Thoughtful left-brain processes can increase life enrichment by helping clinicians rework their life stories into more elevating and enlightening self-narratives. Left-brain strategies can encourage the development of self-compassion and increase meaning in life, which in turn can increase job satisfaction. In contrast to the left-brain strategies that are largely language oriented, logical and effortful, Chapter 9 explores right-brain processes that are predominately visual, intuitive, and effortless. It focuses on the ways in which our lives can be enriched by involvement with art, poetry, and other symbolic activities. In addition, Chapter 9 enforces the importance of self-reflection as foundational for an enriched life and suggests various methods for establishing a self-reflective practice.

Chapter 10 involves the life-enriching effects of creativity. In this discussion, creativity is viewed as an ability that all people can access through combining things or ideas in ways that are novel or useful. Readers are encouraged to embrace their "everyday creativity" as a strategy for maintaining life enrichment. This exploration of creativity is related to the concept of flow and how the flow experience significantly increases life enrichment and personal well-being.

The final chapter of the book summarizes what I believe are three essential results of living an enriched life. The first of these is having a deep well of positive emotions and compassion from which to draw in both personal and professional endeavors. The second effect of living an enriched life is operating with wide margins so that increasingly greater numbers of enriching experiences are encouraged and further enliven the enriched life. The last effect is establishing firm boundaries, derived from a positive view of boundaries. It is based upon the realization that it is not selfish to make one's needs a priority.

All of the information and advice offered in this book is supported by research from various fields including art therapy, psychology, neurology, theology, and ethics. The chapters include practical suggestions for employing the life-enrichment strategies, and it is my hope in providing these suggestions that you are able to have new experiences that enrich your life on an ongoing basis. Finally, each chapter concludes with questions for self-reflection, which when contemplated can deepen personal understanding of the information.

Perils of the Helping Professions   1

Good people are like candles;
they burn themselves up to give others light.
                              Turkish Proverb

I believe that everyone has the capacity to live an enriched and optimally healthy life. However, it has been my observation that in our society, people are more likely to do the opposite of living an enriched life. They have a tendency to work too hard and to sacrifice their physical, mental, and spiritual health. Helping Professionals are especially at risk, due to a focus on assisting others and a pervasive belief that focusing on the self and one's own needs contradicts professional values to care for others. I have encountered this attitude of self-denial among therapists of all kinds, as well as physicians, nurses, and clergy members. However, if Helping Professionals do not take good care of themselves, it is likely that over the long term they will end up ill or disabled with someone else caring for them.

Good self-care efforts can help prevent the development of stress, burnout, and other negative conditions (Kavoor, Mitra, Mahintamani, & Chatterjee, 2015; Malinowski, 2014; Norcross & Guy, 2007). The focus of this book goes beyond self-care; it is not about merely preventing a negative condition or achieving a safe neutral state. The goal of this book it is to bring attention to the topic of life enrichment and to increase understanding of how an enriched life can endow the clinician with a pervasive sense of well-being. Living an enriched life helps people achieve robust physical health, supportive social relationships, meaningful professional work, and an active spiritual life.

This type of holistic health increases vitality and encourages creativity; it imbues the practitioner with the ability to be fully alive and uniquely fulfilled by their professional work.

Working as a psychologist and art therapist in a residential lifestyle medicine program, I have encountered many practitioners of the healing arts who personify the negative effects of constantly focusing outwardly and giving to others; believing that it is selfish to say no, set limits, or take care of themselves. Program participants often lack energy and vitality, and complain of experiencing stress and fatigue. Frequently they state that they eat haphazardly, exercise infrequently, and sleep poorly. Many find themselves in the vicious cycle of drinking caffeine to help them "function" during the day and depending on alcohol to relax in the evening. Often these people tell me that they would consider themselves selfish or self-serving if they thought about their own needs, and especially if they put their own needs above those of their patients or their family members.

A few years ago, I gave a presentation on self-care to a group of art therapists and received a scathing evaluation from an audience member that demonstrates this point. The participant wrote in the comment section, "All this focus on making art for self-care is sickening. Just do the work you signed up for!" I was flabbergasted. I do not know whether this is a common perception among art therapists, but I know that it is a harmful one. People who believe that they should just "get on with the work that they signed up for" likely ignore warning signs in themselves: They work through hunger or physical pain, tension, or depression. In doing so, they may become less effective as healers and their lifespan as a healer may be abbreviated.

Furthermore, someone who identifies as a "helper" may feel uncomfortable with asking for what they need for themselves. In our individualistic society, many people value being good at everything and consider it a weakness to ask for help. However, human beings are social creatures. We function best in groups (couples, families, organizations, and communities) because it is impossible for one person to be good at everything. In a group, people's strengths can be complementary to the strengths of others, and compensate for their weaknesses as well. In reality, it is important for everyone, even those who identify as professional "helpers," to know when to ask for support.

From my perspective, there are three essential pieces to living an enriched life, which will be defined and developed throughout the book: a deep well, wide margins, and firm boundaries. The relationships between these elements and the Life Enrichment Model will be explored and its application in a dynamic balance explained. Living in dynamic balance means that people who live enriched lives know that balance ebbs and flows; it is not static and should not be. Sometimes attention and energy are necessary in one area at other times another area of the LEM is the focus. A deep well of enrichment comes from various aspects of the LEM, but especially from increasing positive emotions like hope, optimism, resiliency, and self-efficacy. To have wide margins is to have time built into the day for a pause. Sometimes this pause is for rest or relaxation and sometimes it is for self-reflection, but it is always necessary to carve out time between activities to live mindfully. In order to embrace firm boundaries, one must realize that it is not selfish to focus on one's own life and heath, but actually a form of necessary self-preservation. When you live an enriched life, you can preserve your health and have more energy to give to others.

Please do not read this book as a list of commandments or things that you "should" be doing or that you have to get right. You are already doing many things right. I would rather that you read the book as an affirmation of what you are already doing to ensure your optimal health. Notice what you are doing already, appreciate it, and perhaps continue doing it with more intention and gratitude. You many also read this book as a list of suggested opportunities to enrich your life in simple but influential ways. Furthermore, I am not seeking to promote a moral imperative that if you feel good you are a good person and vice versa (Cederström & Spicer, 2015). In writing this book, I only want to encourage you to be curious about yourself and the various ways that you can promote the utmost well-being in your life and practice.

There certainly will be times when you feel down or lack motivation; you would not be human if there were not. However, when you live a rich life, it is possible for those dark times to make the light more beautiful. For me, dark times accompanied by dark thoughts occasionally made writing this book extremely difficult. During the dark times, I thought that I could not have anything worthwhile to say to people about wellness if my life were not in perfect balance at all times. A revelation came when I realized that perfectionism was getting in my way. The writing came more easily again when I could tell myself that I do not have to be perfect in order to give advice from my life and my practice. I just have to be honestly striving towards optimal health – and that is how I am living my life.

There has been a great deal of research on the unintended harmful side effects of working in fields where helping others is the primary focus. Many books on self-care discuss the fact that as therapists listen to their clients describe physically or psychologically painful events, they can experience a condition that erodes their physical and mental well-being and interferes with their ability to carry out their work (Kottler, 2017; Malinowski, 2014; Norcross & Guy, 2007; Wicks, 2007). These syndromes, which have been called professional burnout, compassion fatigue, vicarious traumatization, and secondary traumatic stress are characterized by subtle differences but share a great deal of conceptual overlap (Canfield, 2005; Figley & Ludick, 2017; Malinowski, 2014). In fact, the use of various terms to describe these similar conditions may have slowed the progress of research aimed at defining the syndromes. Therefore, the helping professions are delayed in understanding these syndromes, realising their deleterious effects, and describing prevention and treatment efforts (Newell, Nelson-Gardell, & MacNeil, 2016). Readers of this book can remember it is possible to become traumatized by the suffering we encounter as therapists, and that this secondary trauma can cause emotional and physical exhaustion. However, with good self-care practices in place, the enriched life that results offers significant protection against this unintended harm.

Definitions and Distinctions

Professional burnout has been conceptualized as a multidimensional condition resulting from factors related to the helping professional, the populations where the work takes place, and the agency (Newell, et al., 2016). It is the only syndrome that takes organizational factors such as lack of agency resources and support into account (Figley & Ludick, 2017). Interestingly, professional burnout is a term more frequently used in the literature on nurses, physicians, and dentists than other helping professions. Further distinction comes from the fact that burnout is a condition that is a consequence of another syndrome: compassion fatigue, vicarious traumatization, or secondary traumatic stress. Vicarious traumatization and secondary traumatic stress are similar in that they are syndromes that develop due to continuous exposure to client trauma. The definitional difference seems to be that persons suffering from secondary traumatic stress display psychological and physical symptoms in line with Post Traumatic Stress Disorder (PTSD).

According to Malinowski (2014), the symptoms of secondary traumatic stress are very similar to those of PTSD with the exception that whereas the client suffering from PTSD actually has faced a life-threatening event or undergone a serious injury, the clinician suffering from secondary traumatic stress has experienced the trauma secondhand, through attending to client stories of traumatic events and empathizing with their clients' emotions. Vicarious traumatization has been defined as being more highly associated with cognitive changes and beliefs about the world and one's ability to affect change in the world (Newell, et al., 2016).

In the past, compassion fatigue was viewed as a condition with characteristics of both professional burnout and vicarious traumatization (Figley & Ludick, 2017; Newell, et al., 2016) but more recently has been defined as the overall experience of emotional and physical fatigue that can develop in Helping Professionals as a consequence of the chronic use of empathy with those who are suffering (Newell, et al., 2016). In this way, compassion fatigue can be viewed as a consequence of secondary traumatic stress (Figley & Ludick, 2017). The word compassion comes from the Latin roots *pati* and *cum* which together mean "to suffer with" (McNeill, Morrison, & Nouwen, 2006). Compassion is a demanding state of being that requires not only empathy for another's suffering, but also a sense of responsibility for doing something about it. As McNeill, et al. (2016, p. 4) eloquently state:

> Let us not underestimate how hard it is to be compassionate. Compassion is hard because it requires the inner disposition to go with others to places where they are weak, vulnerable, lonely, and broken. But this is not our spontaneous response to suffering. What we desire most is to do away with suffering by fleeing from it or finding a quick cure for it.

This passage fully describes the difficulties of undergoing constant demands on compassion and what the authors state is the most understandable response to suffering: We want to run away from it or quickly patch it up. When it is not possible to flee or fix the ongoing deluge of trauma that Helping Professionals encounter, secondary traumatic stress and compassion fatigue can develop.

Development of Secondary Traumatic Stress and Compassion Fatigue

According to two recent reviews, secondary traumatic stress and compassion fatigue are more likely to develop in Helping Professionals who demonstrate high levels of empathy, prolonged exposure to suffering and high caseloads, low levels of work satisfaction, traumatic memories, and other unexpected life demands (Figley & Ludick, 2017; Turgoose & Maddox, 2017). Although a high level of empathy is a personal characteristic that contributes to a person becoming an effective therapist, it is also one of the factors that leaves counselors vulnerable to developing compassion fatigue or secondary traumatic stress syndrome (Figley & Ludick, 2017; Malinowski, 2014; Turgoose & Maddox, 2017). Empathy and altruism can become depleted as Helping Professionals are continuously confronted with their clients' traumatic experiences, especially if therapists have their own personal history of unresolved trauma. The greater the similarity between the client and therapist trauma, the more likely it is that the therapist will experience secondary traumatic stress and develop compassion fatigue (Figley & Ludick, 2017; Malinowski, 2014).

Other elements contributing to the development of secondary traumatic stress and compassion fatigue are countertransference issues, low levels of work satisfaction, and other life demands (Figley & Ludick, 2017; Malinowski, 2014). Countertransference issues are brought about by unconscious past influences or current life stressors in the therapist that are played out in the therapeutic relationship. For example, a therapist whose father committed suicide might react towards an older, suicidal male client with fear and sadness which interfere with his ability to render successful treatment. When therapists bring internal factors, such as their past or present lives, into their work with clients, countertransference issues become a challenge for both parties.

External factors also can cause Helping Professionals to become dissatisfied at work and contribute to burnout or exacerbate compassion fatigue. Unmanageable caseloads, a lack of respect, job demands that are perceived as out of the person's control and/or a toxic work environment characterized by isolation and a lack of support are work-related external factors that can compound the challenges a therapist may experience in his or her work with clients (Figley & Ludick, 2017; Malinowski, 2014). Personal life stressors such as financial difficulties or changes in personal roles such as care-taking responsibilities can place greater demands on empathic reserves and also contribute to compassion fatigue (Figley & Ludick, 2017).

Prevention and Treatment of Secondary Traumatic Stress and Compassion Fatigue

Despite these challenges to professional well-being and longevity, recent research demonstrates that the development of secondary traumatic stress or compassion fatigue is not inevitable (Figley & Ludick, 2017; Malinowski, 2014; Newell, et al., 2016; Turgoose & Maddox, 2017). It is possible to remain resilient as a Helping Professional and even to develop Post Traumatic Growth (PTG) in response to trauma work. As the name implies, Post Traumatic Growth is a positive condition associated with finding new meaning in life after hardship, viewing the self as resilient and capable, developing a sense of hope for the future, and valuing relationships differently (Bartoskova, 2015; Forgeard, Mecklenburg, Lacasse, & Jayawickreme, 2014; McCormack & Adams, 2016; Želeskov-Dorić, Hedrih, & Dorić, 2012). Factors that contribute to the development of growth rather than professional burnout include maintaining good self-care practices, developing a sense of detachment from professional stressors, having a positive sense of job satisfaction, and acknowledging a strong network of social support. These factors will be fully developed throughout the course of this book to provide you with a comprehensive foundation in life enrichment that can serve to prevent and/or ameliorate secondary traumatic stress and compassion fatigue.

Many Helping Professionals have identified support from compassionate and caring personal relationships as a primary factor in helping them develop resilience in the face of the ongoing stressors of their work (Želeskov-Dorić, et al., 2012). Each of the chapters in this book will emphasize the importance of sharing life enrichment with others as one way to strengthen reserves of positive emotions, empathy, and optimism. In survey research, expert practitioners have described specific professional factors that promoted resilience and prevented burnout in their careers, including having consistent, positive mentor and peer support relationships in the early career phases, having ongoing peer support throughout their career, having multiple professional roles (e.g., teacher, clinician, researcher), and experiencing a health-promoting work environment. Other positive and preventive factors include: dealing directly and openly with professional dilemmas that elicit personal problems, engaging in high quality continuing education, maintaining a balance of solitude and social interactions, investing in a broad array of restorative activities, art making (Salzano, Lindemann, & Tronsky, 2013), and making time for self-reflection (Mullenbach & Skovholt, 2001). Finally, mindfulness strategies have significant preventive effects (Luken & Sammons, 2016; Turgoose & Maddox, 2017). Mindful "micro-self-care practices" can be woven throughout the day to improve mood, decrease emotional reactivity, and increase mind-body awareness (Bush, 2015, p. 5).

Summary and Conclusions

Prolonged exposure to other people's suffering, high levels of empathy, and concern for the welfare and success of their clients can lead Helping

Professionals to develop conditions like vicarious traumatization, secondary traumatic stress, professional burnout, and compassion fatigue. Low work satisfaction, heavy caseloads, lack of support and a personal history of trauma will compound these factors and put certain professionals at higher risk of developing harmful work-related syndromes. However, these factors do not have to inevitably lead to a negative condition. There are many things that therapists can do to prevent or treat debilitating syndromes such as engaging in exceptional self-care practices, fostering supportive social systems, developing routines that encourage detachment from stressful situations, and cultivating a sense of satisfaction in their work. All of these themes and many more will be explored in the next chapters, and their relationships to life enrichment expounded upon.

It was not my wish to begin this book with a chapter on the perils of practicing the helping professions. However, I changed my mind as I was writing the book. I felt that it was necessary to present this cautionary framework so that life-enrichment could be viewed as empowering and not frivolous or superfluous. Self-care is a necessary ethical mandate for those in the helping professions – couching it in the context of life enrichment will hopefully make self-care feel less like another burden competing for your already limited time, and more like a series of consummate supportive practices that can enhance all areas of your life and well-being.

Art Exploration

1. Divide a paper in half and create a two-sided collage that shows the perils and pitfalls of the helping professions on one side and the rewards and potential for growth on the other.
2. Draw or paint a series of three self-portraits that explore the person you were and the factors that influenced your becoming a helping professional, who you are today, and how you would like to look in your optimally healthy future.

Questions for Self-Reflection

1. How do you feel about the level of satisfaction that you achieve from helping others in your current employment situation(s)? Is there any room for improvement? If so, in what areas and how might you go about changing things?

2. Would you rate your current caseload as manageable on most days? Are there days when it feels unmanageable? Do the days when your feelings of manageability and job satisfaction and outnumber those when it does not?
3. Write about the level of personal and professional support that you get from your current employment situation. Is there respect for your position? Are your outcomes valued? Do you have peers, mentors, and supervisors with whom you feel comfortable discussing challenging work situations or clients?
4. Do you have a personal history of trauma that feels unresolved and that could cause a build-up of fear, sadness, or anger that is likely to interfere with your ability to help others and cause secondary traumatic stress and compassion fatigue? If so, please begin your own personal counseling now as you read the rest of the life-enrichment strategies that will improve your overall well-being. A history of personal trauma (any sort of abuse or violence) must be therapeutically addressed for you to be the best person that you can be.

Beyond Self-Care to Life Enrichment   2

The glory of God is man fully alive.

St. Ireaneus (180, p. 4)

Benefits of Life Enrichment

This book is not about expecting to get to neutral or normal; it is about knowing that you can reach beyond the norm to live an enriched life. From a place far above neutral you will have vast stores of energy, confidence, and inspiration to assist others. By living an enriched life you will feel exceptional and demonstrate excellence in all that you do, becoming a confident role model who provides inspiration and motivation for others to live their best lives.

People who live an enriched life are those whose lives are characterized by high levels of happiness and low levels of stress and anxiety. They achieve and maintain a personally defined level of physical vitality and have a curious mind that keeps them actively learning. They are optimally healthy and feel invigorated physically, mentally, socially, and spiritually. By investing in all different forms of their health, this individual feels increased energy and approaches life with a greater capacity to give and receive. This type of invested giving and receiving in relationships and community leads to increased meaning and purpose in their lives. Healthy people living enriched lives are certain that they have significant gifts to give, and convey them in ways that heal the world.

Living an enriched life ensures the development of ingredients essential for being a good caretaker: a deep well, wide margins, and firm boundaries. The deep well is full of psychological resources, physical vitality, and spiritual inspiration. It provides the critical foundation to achieve the depth of empathy necessary to be an excellent therapist. Wide margins ensure time for mindful participation in spiritual practices and self-reflection, and firm boundaries conserve time for personal self-care.

The life of the optimally healthy person will be characterized by "virtuous cycles," not vicious cycles like addiction. A vicious cycle consists of a repetitious set of behaviors in which one difficulty causes another difficulty that worsens the first. In contrast, a virtuous cycle is a cycle of growth where achievement in successive elements in the cycle promotes overall success and well-being (Niemiec, 2014). One good act will engender favorable results and good feelings, which will, in turn, provoke other beneficial behaviors. Therefore, the optimally healthy person demonstrates more good habits and fewer bad habits than someone who is not optimally healthy. Living this way, with a life full of meaning, purpose, and enriching activities, optimally healthy people display lower rates of professional burnout and greater self-rated career satisfaction (Puig, et al., 2012). The Indian mystic and teacher Osho (2002) admonishes us, "The only thing that is in your hands is your life. Make it as rich as possible" (p.14).

When people live enriched lives, they receive stimulating input from many channels: physical, mental, and spiritual. I imagine that they are receiving information from the world in all the ways that God intended them to receive it. I believe that Saint Ireaneus, who lived 2000 years ago, was speaking about this when he wrote the line quoted at the beginning of this chapter: "The glory of God is man fully alive." We are fully alive when we are using all of the faculties that God intended, and that is glorious.

Living an enriched life is one way to promote and maintain optimal health. When people live an enriched life, they are stimulated, animated, and satisfied by many different types of experiences. This intentional richness of input and stimulation means that they are less likely to become stuck in one manner of perceiving themselves or the world, and therefore are more likely to be adaptable and flexible in their approaches to people, problems, and opportunities. An open attitude leads to further life enrichment. Moreover, living an enriched life might be an antidote to the epidemic of stress that is plaguing our nation.

A yearly survey by the American Psychological Association revealed that two-thirds of Americans regard themselves as somewhat to very stressed about the future, finances, or work (American Psychological Association

(APA), 2017). The survey also showed that more people than ever reported physical or emotional symptoms of stress in the previous month, including headaches, depression, and anxiety. Survey participants endorsed many positive coping mechanisms such as performing physical exercise, listening to music, and engaging in meditation; but the majority (56%) reported that they could use more skills and support than they currently have to deal with the stress in their lives (APA, 2017). In addition, many people use maladaptive coping mechanisms such as overeating or drinking alcohol when faced with stress (APA, 2017; Holton, Barry, & Chaney, 2016) and a percentage of those individuals go on to become addicted.

In a fascinating series of experiments on addiction, Dr. Bruce Alexander and his colleagues challenged the prevailing belief in the early 1980s that mere exposure to heroin was enough to cause addiction to it. In a typical experiment, laboratory rats were placed in standard wire cages and given a choice of opiate-infused water or regular water to drink. The majority became addicted, disregarding the plain water and taking in drugs to the point of death. But these results gave Dr. Alexander pause. Upon reflection, he thought that if he were a rat in a boring wire cage, he would probably become addicted also; there was nothing else to do in the uninteresting environment. However, he hypothesized that if rats lived in an enriched environment they would not choose the drugged water. So, Dr. Alexander and his colleagues conducted a series of experiments in which they provided one group of rats with a large enclosure that was supplied with structures to explore, toys to play with, and other rats to interact with; the enclosure became known as Rat Park. Other groups of rats lived in the standard wire cages and all were provided with a choice between opiate-infused and regular water.

Through this series of experiments, the research group demonstrated that the majority of rats who had the chance to "change their cages" and live an enriched life in the Rat Park did not become addicted (Alexander, 2010). Other investigators have replicated the studies to further demonstrate the positive effects of an enriched environment on reducing the propensity for addiction (Deehan, Palmatier, Cain, & Kiefer, 2011; Galaj, Manuszak, & Ranaldi, 2016). Further, even short-term exposure to an enriched environment has a stress-reducing effect on the brain and body. This is why we return from a vacation feeling refreshed and reinvigorated (Ashokan, Hegde, & Mitra, 2016). The long-term benefits of life enrichment are even greater and longer lasting than the short-term effects of a holiday.

The premise of this book is that in the short and long term, living an enriched life is a superior way for everyone to live. Living an enriched life fills the deep well of positive emotions and compassion that can make people more empathetic community members. An enriched life also creates greater openness to helping others in meaningful ways. Moreover, life enrichment increases genuine generosity and safeguards health practitioners against developing burnout.

Definition of Optimal Health

When I write about optimal health, I am referring to a life that is characterized by physical, mental, social, and spiritual well-being. I have learned through my work in lifestyle medicine that people who are optimally healthy have robust physical health, engaging social relationships, a stimulating work life, and a nourishing spiritual life. By robust physical health, I mean that people are strong and capable, perhaps even exceeding age expectations for strength and ability. Robustly healthy people also are agile and flexible and have well-supported immune functioning. By engaging social relationships, I mean that people have a circle of intimate family members and friends who are emotionally available and supportive, share common interests and values, and who provide intellectual stimulation. Optimally healthy people have friends or family members in their lives that they could call at any hour of the day or night for help and support. In addition, they have a circle of close friends and a larger circle of acquaintances that support their physical, intellectual, and spiritual growth. The community where optimally healthy people live supports their physical well-being.

Optimally healthy people have a stimulating work life; they have a passion for their work that makes it feel enlivening rather than draining. People with a stimulating occupation believe that their work goes beyond "doing a job" or "having a career" to having a calling (Kelley & Kelley, 2013; Smith, 2016). Their daily work stretches the limits of their knowledge and pushes them towards constant innovation and improvement. At the same time, they are able to master their work challenges for optimal results, often achieving a state of "flow" (Csikszentmihalyi, 2008). People with a stimulating work life feel that that their unique strengths and abilities are utilized and appreciated. They grow through their work: They set definite goals for themselves and attempt various problem-solving strategies to meet their goals. They evaluate problem-solving strategies, alter them if necessary, and re-implement those that are most effective. Although challenged they can achieve a state of flow in which they feel completely absorbed in their work; they are capable, masterful, and satisfied by a job well done (Csikszentmihalyi, 2008).

Finally, optimally healthy people have an active and nourishing spiritual life which provides purpose and meaning. A strong spiritual sense enriches life with meaning and promotes well-being. In writing about "spirituality," I am referring to the broad definition of spiritual which stems from the Latin root word *respire* or "to breathe." Optimally healthy people feel that their life is guided by a force that breathes life into them (Hinz, 2006). They live with a sense of purpose greater than themselves that informs their life and gives them day-to-day vigor, along with bursts of energy for exceptional activities. Following their purpose gives life meaning beyond merely making a living. People with an active spiritual life feel called to serve others but not at the expense of their own health.

Summary and Conclusions

One aim of this book is to help readers understand how an enriched life provides a pervasive sense of well-being and to demonstrate how it prevents the development of stress, anxiety, and other negative conditions. Life enrichment means that people take in experiences from the world in all of the ways that life has to offer: physically, mentally, socially, and spiritually. When people appreciate and develop the richness and depth life presents, they are more likely to be optimally healthy and therefore the best possible Helping Professionals. It is my hope that this book will stimulate self-reflection and robust self-care efforts. It is full of practical suggestions that can be shared with friends, family members, and clients.

As I described in Chapter 1, whenever I give presentations on self-care there is inevitably an undercurrent of fear that people will become "selfish" in thinking about or doing so much for themselves. However, I believe that we are being selfish if we do not take care of ourselves. When Helping Professionals continuously sacrifice their own well-being to care for others, resentment grows and soon they are giving grudgingly rather than generously. The building resentment means that unmet needs are in the background of each interaction and bitterness often seeps into the foreground. In attempting to avoid feeling selfish, the therapist who operates without limits can become a prisoner of his or her own unmet needs – these needs driving interactions without their awareness.

In my opinion, the foundation of an exceptional professional practice is living a deeply enriched life, which includes regular attention to meeting one's own needs. Exquisitely fulfilling one's own needs results in optimal health. From this vantage point, Health Professionals are confident in their abilities and also in the fact that their lives can serve as a template for clients to emulate. The ingredients essential for being a good caretaker are the products of living an enriched life: a deep well of psychological resources, physical vitality, and spiritual inspiration, wide margins for mindful self-reflection, and firm boundaries to ensure time for effective personal self-care. To develop all of these elements and allow them to thrive in the context of an enriched life, it is imperative to know that self-care is not self-indulgent – it is treating yourself like you would treat other people. Put yourself and your needs on the list (and maybe even at the top of the list) of priorities. Remember, self-care is not selfish, it is self-preservation.

Suggestions for Art Reflection

1. Draw your own "Rat Park." What would your ideal environment include to make it optimally stimulating and enriching for you?
2. Create an image of a deep well, wide margins, or firm boundaries. Include in your image how you believe these elements will help you be the best possible helping professional that you can be.

Questions for Self-Reflection

1. What is your position on self-care and the importance of self-care as a therapist?
2. What sorts of self-care activities do you regularly engage in?
3. How can you honor the self-care activities that you already perform as life enrichment, beyond self-care? Would your practices have to be altered in any way to do so?

The Life Enrichment Model   3

*There is no knowledge so hard to acquire
as the knowledge of how to live this life well and naturally.*
                              Michel de Montaigne (1999, p. 193)

The Life Enrichment Model (LEM) is a representation of human functioning that comprises how the brain and body take in and are affected by various life experiences. As such, the LEM can provide a structure to envision the enriched life. The Life Enrichment Model is an adaptation of the Expressive Therapies Continuum (ETC), which is a theoretical framework from the art therapy literature. The ETC was originally designed to explain how individuals take in and process information in their interactions with a range of art materials and processes. It is a theory that describes how and why different forms of artistic media and instruction have psychologically therapeutic effects (Kagin and Lusebrink, 1978; Lusebrink, 1990; 2014). The ETC theory was extended to a systems approach that explained the various ways that all of the expressive arts can have therapeutic benefits (Lusebrink, 1991). This book represents an extension and adaptation of the ETC to general life experiences. I have used the ETC as a starting point in conceptualizing the ways that people can enrich their lives, and the adapted version or Life Enrichment Model (LEM) is displayed in Figure 3.1.

The LEM offers a way to conceptualize and practically create an enriched life, one that will help foster optimal health and allow therapists to cultivate resiliency, invest more deeply in their professional practice, and achieve a satisfying balance between their personal and professional lives. Similar to

18 The Life Enrichment Model

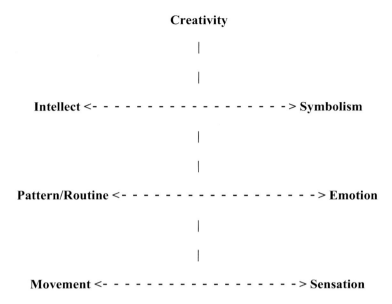

Figure 3.1 The Life Enrichment Model (LEM): A Pathway to Optimal Health

the Expressive Therapies Continuum, the LEM might be seen as a schematic diagram of the brain and how we interact in the world to process information. This diagram represents different levels of brain functioning from simple to complex as well as left and right hemisphere functioning (Lusebrink, 2004; 2010; 2014). The diagram in Figure 3.1 shows the structure of the LEM, from rudimentary movement and sensual functioning on the bottom to the most sophisticated forms of information processing at the intellect and symbolism level at the top of the structure.

Movement and Sensation

Information processing begins at the Kinesthetic/Sensory level of the ETC. This kind of brain activity corresponds to what some have called the reptilian brain (MacLean, 1985). Structures like the cerebellum, basal ganglia, primary motor cortex and sensorimotor cortex represent the evolutionarily oldest structures of the brain, those that do not require conscious thought in mediating behavior. Human beings do not have to think through the process of walking in order to put one foot in front of another. They do not have to engage in conscious thought in order to mediate sensory experiences and initiate automatic behaviors. If I place my hand on a hot stove, consciously thinking, "That stove is hot, I should move my hand" would take a few seconds. I would receive a third degree burn if I took that long to process the sensory stimulation. Instead, I react immediately based on what I experience: The sensation initiates action. It is adaptive and life-saving for all species to respond to noxious or dangerous stimuli without using slow and deliberate conscious thought, as well as to perform automatic behaviors like walking. The lack of conscious thought involved in the processing of movement and sensation information is what defines the reptilian brain.

The Kinesthetic/Sensory level of the ETC is analogous to the oldest brain structures, and also represents the most developmentally basic (youngest) manner in which humans process information. This is the way that infants and toddlers take in, process, and express information (Piaget, 2000). Infants make many random movements that produce different kinds of stimulation. As they get a little older, babies begin to purposely recreate movements associated with pleasant sensory stimuli and avoid those paired with unpleasant sensations. This rudimentary learning takes place through movement and sensation. All people must use sensorimotor learning on a regular basis when adapting to their physical environment or when learning a new physical skill (Wolpert, Diedrichsen, & Flanagan, 2011). However, because it is largely used without conscious thought, sensorimotor learning is frequently underappreciated.

The movement/sensation level of the Life Enrichment Model is perhaps the most neglected avenue of information processing and experience in our 21st century Western society. In fact, people are taught to not pay attention to the wisdom of bodily sensations. They are told to ignore pain. The adage, "no pain, no gain" encourages people to push through painful physical sensations in order to train their bodies to perform better. However, most of us know that if we persist in a workout despite being in pain, we will likely do damage to muscles or joints. Many people engage in purposeful physical activity through exercise and recreation, but ignore their physical needs and sensations as they perform sedentary jobs and then sit to "relax" once they return home from work. A tendency to avoid physical sensation and physical signals could contribute to a tendency to overwork and to burn out. Chapters 4 and 5 of his book will suggest different avenues to increase the enjoyment of movement and sensation in life.

Sensuality can enrich your life when you notice and delight in the beautiful sights around you, luxuriate in the sensual aspects of touch, relish sumptuous tastes and aromas, and make sure that you appreciate silence as well as sounds that you enjoy. Engaging in regular physical exercise is a powerful part of living an enriched life. Regular physical exercise reduces stress, helps maintain weight, improves sleep, increases relaxation and alertness, and improves cognitive functioning and mood. Sensuality and movement are the physical foundation for the deep well of positive psychological resources, physical vitality, and spirituality that not only helps avoid mental and physical exhaustion, but also boosts one's quality of life far above the norm.

Routine and Emotion

Chapter 6 discusses the next level of sophistication in brain functioning, represented by structures called the limbic system or the mammalian brain (MacLean, 1985). The limbic structures of the brain give mammals the ability to analyze patterns in their environment for similarities and discrepancies, and to respond to those patterns with corresponding emotional indicators. Pattern similarities confirm the status quo; the surroundings are satisfactory and no emotional signal is generated. Pattern discrepancies – differences in line, shape, color, and pattern – cause new structures to stand out from the background into the foreground. Unexpected incongruities elicit emotional signals. Moreover, if an animal or human breaks routine and behaves unexpectedly, members of the community are alerted or distressed by this change in expected or patterned behavior. This distress prompts new forms of behavior in the witness as she or he responds to the unfamiliar. Therefore, the limbic system functions as an intermediary between urgent messages from the environment and action in the environment.

Each of the six primary emotions (anger, sadness, fear, happiness, interest/ surprise, and disgust) functions as a potentially lifesaving signal of threat or opportunity (Ekman, 2007). The most commonly discussed example of an emotional signal is that of fear. Fear is a signal of the presence of a threat in the environment. It signals the animal or person to freeze, flee, fight, or faint in order to save its life (Bracha, 2004; Ekman, 2007). The five other primary emotions function in a similar way – they indicate the presence of either threat or opportunity and encourage action to preserve life. Although the physical existence of most people in our Western society is not threatened on a daily basis, we still maintain the ability to analyze the patterns of our environment, develop comforting routines, and send and receive emotional signals.

It is popularly believed that emotions are evolutionarily conserved indicators of threat or opportunity that once played a deep role in our ability to survive. They are believed to be "hard wired" into people of every culture, identifiable by specific facial expressions from infancy onwards. However, new research shows that learning, both personal and cultural, influences our perceptions of emotion much more that originally believed (Feldman Barrett, 2017). One aspect of living an enriched life is to learn to respond intentionally rather than automatically in response to emotional signals. Chapters 6 and 7 in this book will focus on how this level of information processing helps preserve our relationships.

Intellect and Symbolism

The cerebral cortex, or the "human brain," is the final layer of the brain addressed. This is where the most sophisticated forms of information processing, available only to human beings, take place (MacLean, 1985). This complex thought is characterized in the left hemisphere by effortful, linear, logical, and language-oriented processes. The sophisticated functions of the cerebral cortex, and in particular of the prefrontal cortex, support cause and effect thinking, planning, and delayed gratification. This type of thinking is uniquely human and allows people to plan a course of action, work through the potential consequences of decisions before they take action, and adds to life enrichment as people deliberately learn new things. These ways of thinking are contrasted with right-hemisphere processes, which are more likely to be holistic, visual-spatial, spiritual, and intuitive. This complex right brain-influenced thought allows for life enrichment through the arts, metaphor, and ritual. Chapters 8 and 9 will present information on how to enrich your life through both types of sophisticated cognitive processes.

Creativity

The Creative level of the Life Enrichment Model, like that of the ETC, emphasizes "putting it all together" and the self-actualizing tendencies of the human being (Lusebrink, 1990). Engaging in creative activity involves coordinated activation of many brain structures. In proposing the LEM, I would like to combine this definition of creative functioning with the definition of creativity that many psychologists use, which is, putting things or ideas together in ways that are novel and useful (Runco & Jaeger, 2012). This definition of creativity is inclusive and emphasizes the fact that everyone is creative in different ways. All people should be encouraged to embrace their "everyday creativity" (Richards, 2014); because living creatively enhances personal growth, it encourages people to move beyond their defensiveness to express aspects of their highest selves (Richards, 2014). Chapter 10 will encourage exploration and celebration of everyday creativity. When we are in love with life and all of its creative possibilities we are living an enriched life.

The Life Enrichment Model can help summarize the various ways that the brain and body take in, process, and express information and provide a structure for life enrichment. It suggests that the more enriched one's life becomes, the more likely they are to be in dynamic balance and optimally healthy. It is important to remember that there is no pressure to engage in one activity from every component of the LEM on a daily basis. Living an enriched life should not become a source of stress or a burdensome obligation. As long as there is flexible and changing balance among the various components over the course of a couple of weeks, life can be optimally enriched.

Balance in life is not a static endpoint to be achieved and then forgotten. I have used the term dynamic balance to reinforce the fact that life elements are constantly in motion and a good balance can look different each week. The optimally functioning person can move easily and adaptively between ways of responding in the world represented by the LEM components. Further, the components of the LEM can organize life enrichment efforts and provide a springboard for intentional action. The balanced person is able to take in and process information with all of the LEM components, and actively seeks out experiences with a wide variety of modalities to engage in intentional life enrichment.

Intentional Enrichment

There is a difference between living a life that is purposefully enriched and one that is packed full of activities. People who overschedule and overcommit themselves, without making time to pause and reflect, usually do not take the time to notice the enriching effects of all the things that they are doing. They are busy and overburdened. However, most people already participate in some life-enriching self-care efforts, and a first step should be recognizing and celebrating what people already do to take care of themselves. Next, it is important to critically assess how these activities are working.

You can use the circular form provided in Figure 3.2 below as a template to help you figure out how you are doing in the various areas of life enrichment. The circle is divided into six equal parts, each representing one

The Life Enrichment Model   23

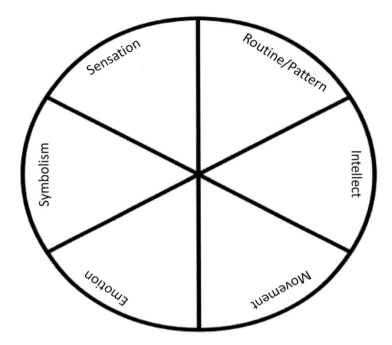

Figure 3.2 Life Enrichment Model Circle Assessment

aspect of the LEM. You may color or decorate (with symbols drawn or cut from a magazine) these areas, as you understand them so far, to show how much time per week you spend in each pursuit. When you are finished, tuck the image away in the first part of this book to review at a later time.

After completing this assessment, use the questions at the end of this chapter to reflect on the practices that you already cultivate to care for yourself, honor those that really work, and drop some that are no longer effective. Only then should you try to supplement, with purpose and intention, areas that need to be balanced. The aim of this book is not to give you another set of rules to live by or to add a long "to do list" to your life. Rather, its purposes are to help you take inventory of your self-care practices, add information about potential activities, and help you understand that balance among all of the ways that information is processed and expressed is optimal. This book should help you take stock of your life and intentionally enhance areas that are ignored or sometimes neglected.

Dynamic Balance

The same bidirectional relationship between opposite poles of each level of the Expressive Therapies Continuum (Kagin & Lusebrink 1978; Lusebrink, 1990) exists between the two components on each level of the Life Enrichment Model. This means that as involvement with activities on one side of the model (Movement/Sensation; Pattern/Emotion; Intellect/Symbolism) increases, one's ability to be occupied with the other side of the level is decreased. This is neither positive nor negative; it is just a fact to notice as you think about refining your self-care practices: They influence one another, they are not static, and sometimes in combination, they work best. For example, on the first level, as you become more vigorously physically active, your ability to perceive fine sensations diminishes. On the second level, involvement with pattern and routine is one way to decrease emotional responding. Finally, with the third level, the concentration involved with left-hemisphere processes reduces the likelihood of intuitive flashes of insight. In general, a dynamic balance between the components is sought so that the ability to fluidly move between ways of responding in the world is manifest. The last chapters will demonstrate how knowledge of this relationship can be used to deliberately choose complementary experiences to provide optimal life enrichment.

Summary and Conclusions

The Life Enrichment Model (LEM) grew out of my commitment to the Expressive Therapies Continuum and how this theory explains the therapeutic aspects of art making. Moving beyond art to the larger realm of activities and life experiences, the LEM provides a structure for conceptualizing and objectively creating an enriched life. The model takes into account the various ways that the brain and body process information – physically, emotionally, and intellectually – and as such will provide a way to assess life enrichment efforts and amend them if necessary.

This chapter emphasized that the various LEM components operate in conjunction with one another and that balance among components is not fixed but flexible. In fact, if life enrichment efforts become too fixed, they lose their effectiveness. Many people do not realize that self-care practices have to be many and varied to maintain potency. The LEM suggests that intentional enrichment will move you beyond self-care to living a life of robust, optimal health. The remainder of this book will examine the components of the LEM in detail and provide practical suggestions for enrichment.

Questions for Self-Reflection

1. Did the circle that you created and colored reflect a balanced and enriched life, as you currently understand it?
2. In what area(s) of the Life Enrichment Model do you have confidence that you are living an enriched life?
3. Does your life contain practices that you thought were enriching but with further reflection no longer seem to be?
4. What area(s) of the Life Enrichment Model need to be developed or augmented?

Life Enrichment through Sensation

4

> *True silence is the rest of the mind, and is to the spirit what sleep is to the body, nourishment and refreshment.*
> William Penn (1726, p. 899)

When writing about sensation, I refer to the awareness of a particular feeling or effect that the body experiences due to the stimulation of a sense organ. There are many ways that using the five senses can be life enriching: eating sumptuous food and sipping enticing drink, inhaling enveloping aromas, and luxuriating the physical sensations of touch. According to Maria Montessori, who spent her life studying childhood education, the foundation of learning is in exercising the senses. Sensory information plays a vital role in attracting and focusing attention, engendering concentrated learning efforts, and providing enjoyment to enhance persistence. Montessori believed that sensory stimulation was necessary to move learning from concrete to abstract (Montessori, 1967).

In the Life Enrichment Model, sensory information is a foundation for life enrichment. It inspires awe and increases psychological, emotional, and physical well-being (Rudd, Vohs, & Aaker, 2012; Stellar, et al., 2015). Sensual experiences evoke beauty, awe, and joy, which contribute to the deep well of positive emotions, satisfaction, and compassion that characterizes an enriched life. In addition, the practice of noticing sensory input grounds people in the present moment and increase mindfulness. Being in the moment with sensory experiences can alter the subjective experience of time and encourage living with wide margins (Rudd, et al., 2012).

Olfactory Sensation

The world is full of natural aromas that can increase energy and mood or decrease arousal and promote calm. From time immemorial men and women have taken advantage of the mood-altering effects of aroma. There is evidence of the use of essential oils made from fragrant plants for medicinal purposes in ancient Egypt, Greece, Rome, India, and China (Aftel, 2014). There is a great deal of anecdotal evidence and increasing scientific proof that demonstrates the effectiveness of various aromas. Peppermint is known as a physically enlivening scent and cinnamon as one that provides intellectual stimulation (Lobel, 2014). Lavender, almond, and jasmine are calming aromas; frankincense has been promoted for its antidepressant properties (Aftel, 2014). Lemon increases positive mood (Kiecolt-Glaser, et al., 2008). Aroma has been used as a complementary therapy for such things as pain relief (Bagheri-Nesami, et al., 2014) stress reduction (Chen, Fang, & Fang, 2015; Hur, Song, Lee, & Lee, 2014; Redstone, 2015; Tang & Tse, 2014), and sleep enhancement (Hwang & Shin, 2015; Lillehei & Halcon, 2014; Lytle, Mwatha, & Davis, 2014).

The most rigorous scientific studies of aroma have been conducted on the effects of lavender. Although researchers have used different substances (actual plants, essential oils) and delivery methods, a handful of studies have provided increasing evidence that the scent of lavender can effectively decrease perceptions of pain (Sasannejad, et al., 2012) and stress (Hur, et al., 2014), as well as improve sleep (Hwang & Shin, 2015; Lytle, Mwatha, & Davis, 2014). Despite the growing body of evidence supporting the therapeutic effects of lavender, researchers criticize that expectations might be more influential than aroma in reducing stress or increasing relaxation (Howard & Hughes, 2008).

Even if expectation more than aroma is the agent of change, there are still many ways in which life can be enriched with fragrance. After selecting a fragrance with the desired relaxing or uplifting properties, the aroma can be distributed using a room diffuser for an all-round effect. Scented candles can give a warm, subtle aroma to a room. Aroma can be worn on the body through scented soaps, creams, and perfumes. Do not overlook the opportunity to infuse daily tasks with new properties by choosing dish soap and laundry detergent wisely. Enjoy the way that the warm water enhances the aroma of thoughtfully chosen soap to make the dishwashing experience thoroughly enjoyable. Remember that it is not necessary to go out and buy new products, but use the ones that you have mindfully. Make sure to pause and notice their effects.

Sharing Aroma

One interesting study demonstrated that stimulating scents like peppermint promoted an exclusionary state, whereas the use of relaxing aromas, such as lavender, enhanced interpersonal inclusion (Sellaro, Hommel, Rossi Paccani, & Colzato, 2015). These results indicate that relaxing aromas are better for sharing with others to increase closeness. The use of perfume is one way that aroma is shared to enhance relationships (Aftel, 2014). By developing a personal scent, people augment the pleasure of being around loved ones. Sharing scented flowers or the heady aroma of wine also heightens feelings in intimate relationships.

Visual Sensation

The effects of visual cues are well known to product designers, marketers, and advertisers who use the psychological properties of various colors and shapes to influence consumer choice. Art therapists value various materials for the visual effects they produce. In addition, there are physical and psychological benefits to surrounding oneself with beauty and appreciating things that are beautiful (Ferrucci, 2009). It is possible to enrich one's environment with color and art and to increase appreciation of nature and beauty in all forms. One can take advantage of the soothing or stimulating properties of color. Simply put, high-arousal colors are those on the long end of the wavelength spectrum: red, orange, and yellow. These colors tend to make the heart beat faster; they cause physiological arousal. On the opposite end of the color spectrum, green, blue, and violet are known as low-arousal colors. They tend to promote feelings of calm by lowering heart rate and blood pressure (Alter, 2014; Sakuragi & Sugiyama, 2011). The effects of low- and high-arousal colors should be kept in mind when decorating homes or offices; color sets the tone that will provide the desired energy level.

Artistic touches in houses or offices might excite or calm at first, but those effects wear off after a while. This is because people habituate to anything that they see too often, even beautiful things (Ferrucci, 2009). Therefore, to maintain the relaxing or galvanizing effects of decorative touches, it will be necessary to change them every now and then. Merely changing the location of a painting will make it new again. The same effect can occur with vases, pillows, and other decorations. In fact, some people regularly change furniture arrangements to create interest or seasonally change pillows, tablecloths, and throw rugs. This type of rearranging is one way to make sure that people "see" the beauty of their homes again and experience the relaxing or exciting properties anew.

Environmental enrichment also can come about through spending time in naturally beautiful surroundings. Studies have demonstrated that spending time in nature reduces stress and improves mood compared to spending time in an urban environment (Li, 2018; Louv, 2011). Many of the people whom I interviewed in the course of writing this book described time spent in nature as rejuvenating, healing, calming, and fortifying. They looked forward to time in nature on the weekends to recharge themselves after long days at work. Appreciating natural surroundings means taking time to view the sunset, the moonrise, and the constellations in the night sky. These experiences also can fill one with a sense of awe that increases feelings of subjective wellbeing (Rudd, et al., 2012). Simply including houseplants in your décor or having a window with a view of nature have been shown to reduce stress (Louv, 2011; Ratey & Manning, 2015). Even those who are housebound can benefit from the beauty of bringing nature indoors through the use of flowers and houseplants (Dijkstra, Pieters, & Pruyn, 2008) as well as appreciating views from the window. A Hindu saying, quoted by Joseph Campbell in *The Power of Myth*, emphasizes that being in the presence of natural beauty can even connect you with the divine: "When, before the beauty of a sunset or a mountain, you pause and exclaim, "Ah," you are participating in divinity" (p. 258).

Helping Professionals take note: If you have a window with a view, make sure to take time each day to enjoy it. Add a houseplant to your office to take advantage of the stress-relieving properties of being around nature. Three plants that will grow in artificial light (with no natural sunlight) are golden pathos, peace lily, and sliver queen. Make sure to water sparingly in these conditions (perhaps once a month to begin with) and do not disrupt them by repotting more often than every two years.

Sharing Beauty

It is possible to enhance the power of pleasing visual stimulation by sharing it with loved ones. People find that their relationships grow stronger and deeper when they appreciate beauty together. Some would say that the presence of others is what makes the experience of beauty possible (Ferrucci, 2009). Walking or hiking with someone is one way to share and expand the effects of visual beauty. Posting beautiful photographs on Snapchat, Instagram, or Facebook is a common way that people share the beauty that they encounter each day and thus multiply its effects as they receive positive feedback. The effects of online sharing are even more powerful if the sharing is targeted and personal. The experience of appreciating beauty could be greatly enhanced if a photograph was taken and shared with one person specifically in mind. This type of photograph, sent with a message conveying "this beautiful scene made me think of you," could be considered part of "the work of love" that enriches lives.

Tactile Sensation

Life enrichment through tactile sensation involves being aware of the sensual aspects of the fabrics and surfaces in work and home environments. The fabric that clothing is made of can be soft, supportive, and comforting. On the other hand, clothing can be too warm, too tight, or scratchy. Although a relatively minor irritation, inappropriate clothing can be a significant source of stress. Through awareness of clothing, we can ensure that it has a soothing and not irritating effect throughout the day. Likewise, the surfaces where people work can be an irritant if they are too cold or hard. Often people rest their wrists on the cool surfaces of desks or computers as they pause in their typing. These cold surfaces could contribute to the development of carpal tunnel syndrome; to increase wellness people can use a warm, soft gel pad to lift their wrists off cold, hard surfaces when using the computer mouse. Furthermore, ergonomically designed furniture can provide life enrichment and promote good health. People can make sure that the chairs that they sit in and the desk where they work are well designed and fitting. Proper fit can reduce the likelihood of neck and back problems later.

Sharing Touch

Tactile sensation can include all types of positive, soothing, and healing touches. Through various forms of person-to-person contact such as hugs and massage, oxytocin, a hormone that acts as a neurotransmitter, is released in the brain. This leads to feelings of interpersonal liking or loving, warmth, and bonding. The interpersonal effects of human touch and the neurotransmitters involved might be on the crest of the next treatments for addiction (Bowen & Neumann, 2017). A 20-second hug can counteract the effects of stress that have built up during the day, and a 30-minute massage can alleviate those that have built up over the course of the week.

Taste Sensation

Experiencing the intense flavors of high-quality food is life enriching. This was the subject of Peter Kaminsky's book, *Culinary Intelligence*. Kaminsky is a former food critic and cookbook author who discovered that he could significantly influence his health outcomes and increase his enjoyment of food by "investing in flavor per calorie." He explained that by choosing to eat fresh, locally grown, organic food, his greater monetary investment in groceries paid off by allowing him to eat smaller quantities of extremely flavorful fare. He found that when flavor was intense, it took less food to feel satisfied. In addition, by investing in flavor per calorie, Kaminsky (2013) significantly reduced his weight and lowered his risk of diabetes and other health problems. By focusing on flavor, anyone will find that eating can be considered "dining," and dining can be an enriching experience.

The freshest alternatives for flavorful foods are available at local farmers' markets. People might also choose a community supported agriculture (CSA) initiative. A CSA usually offers a box of locally grown vegetables and fruit (occasionally these boxes offer organic eggs and meat products) delivered to a central pickup location or individual homes. One advantage of a CSA is that people try products that they would not normally buy and many offer weekly recipe ideas for box contents. It is important to vary food intake, because eating the same foods all the time restricts the nutrients received and leads to flavor dilution. Repeatedly eating the same foods reduces taste stimulation, which can mean that people end up eating larger quantities when what they really want is diversity of taste sensation. Eating different foods is life enriching.

Mindful eating also increases the flavor experience and helps people appreciate being hungry (Chozen Bays, 2009). In addition, mindful eating helps people understand that there are many different types of hunger. Living a fast-paced life, people often do not slow down to realize what they are truly hungry for – they reach for food when they notice a need because food is ubiquitous and easy. There are at least seven different types of hunger: "eye hunger" for visually pleasing sights; "mouth hunger" for various sensations like crunchy and smooth; "nose hunger" for aromatic substances; "mind hunger" for intellectual stimulation; "heart hunger" for emotional soothing; "stomach hunger" to fill an empty stomach; and body hunger to nourish our cells (Chozen Bays, 2009). Food reliably and appropriately satisfies stomach hunger and body hunger; the other types of hunger are better gratified through other means. When people live mindlessly, they often rely on food to assuage all types of hunger. Living more mindfully, and especially living an enriched life, you will notice a variety of experiences that meet your important needs.

After learning about life enrichment through sensation, a client brought me the bouquet of heirloom roses shown in Plate 1 to demonstrate that she understood the concept. These unusually colored flowers enriched both of our lives through the viewing and sharing of sensation.

Sharing Flavor

Sharing meals with friends and family is a way to appreciate unique and pleasing flavors, but it also has a vast range of emotional benefits. A majority of scientific studies performed over the last twenty years support the fact that when families eat meals together, children of all ages fare better physically, emotionally, and academically. Regardless of family structure – single parent, step-family, or traditional family – children of families who eat meals together show benefits in improved school grades, reduced risky behavior, and better eating habits. Children who eat dinner with their families are less likely to be overweight, chose unhealthy foods, and demonstrate disordered eating. They are more likely to eat fruits and vegetables. Adolescents in families who share meals are less likely to smoke cigarettes, drink alcohol, use marijuana, and engage in premarital sex. The effects of family meals are not always related to feelings of closeness in the family, but probably are due to talking about the day, sharing stories and emotions, and the active problem solving that takes place both in gaining feedback about stories and negotiating family "air time." Eating together has been shown to have long-lasting protective effects against the development of substance abuse for girls. In one study, young women who ate dinner with their families as teenagers were less likely to abuse substances five years later (Fishel, 2015; Meier & Musick, 2014).

Auditory Sensation and Silence

We live in a time where we are constantly assailed by auditory stimulation; the television provides background noise, we listen to music or podcasts through earbuds as we exercise or the news on the radio as we drive. Whether we want it to or not, music accompanies us in grocery stores, shopping malls, and doctors' offices. All of this auditory stimulation can be a day-to-day irritation. There is evidence that moments of silence can reduce autonomic nervous system arousal and stress (Bernardi, Porta, & Sleight, 2006). Silence can replenish mental resources and encourage creativity (Kagge, 2017; Kelley & Kelley, 2013). Most surprising to researchers, silence can promote the growth of new brain cells in laboratory mice (Kirste, et al., 2015). This surprising effect was discovered in a study where silence was supposed to be the control or neutral condition, but actually was demonstrated to be a powerful intervention in itself. Silence is healing.

Therefore, the first thing that people can do to enrich their lives in an auditory way is not additive, but subtractive. People can try to reduce the noise in their lives that they have control over because some – from traffic, air conditioning or heating systems, and appliances – is unavoidable. It is possible to schedule the use of some appliances like the dishwasher for times that people are out of the house. Replace older appliances with quieter versions as needed. Double or triple pane windows can reduce traffic noise. It is important to be judicious about when the television is turned on and try being in silence. Carefully chosen music can set a mood or provide other desired effects.

Listening to music has many enriching effects on body, mind, and spirit. A discussion of the myriad beneficial effects of creating music and rhythm is beyond the scope of this book; this section will focus merely on the effects of listening to music. Music can evoke powerful emotions and motivate. It can enhance mood and increase feelings of happiness. Studies have shown that listening to one's favorite music can reduce subjective ratings of anxiety as well as objective measures of stress such as blood pressure (Dobek, Beynon, Bosma, & Stroman, 2014; Garcia & Hand, 2016; Hsieh, et al., 2014; Lesiuk, 2008). Listening to music can reduce the perception of pain, and studies even suggest that listening to classical music can boost immune functioning (Jha, et al., 2015). So, there are many ways that listening to music can enrich your life.

Sharing Music

Sharing music can enrich a romantic partnership because couples often bond with the help of shared songs. These preferences might endure because they emphasize shared values and commemorate special times. Music connects church families through shared hymns. Shared music bonds countries and communities through national anthems and traditional songs. In addition, mothers and daughters who enjoy shared musical choices report more harmonious relationships (Morgan, MacDonald, & Pitts, 2015).

Sensuality and the Brain

There are many benefits of using art in ways that emphasize its sensual aspects. Using art, people can be immersed in tactile or visual sensation as a way to feel centered and calm. The rhythmic stroking of clay, for example, can slow down the thoughts that seem to continuously crowd people's minds, allowing for a time of focused calm. Research in the neuroscience of human experience demonstrates that several large-scale brain networks dominate brain functioning; the two most applicable here are the Default Mode Network (DMN) and the Direct Experience Network (DEN). Functional magnetic resonance imaging (fMRI) studies show that when people are not active, meaning they are daydreaming, the medial prefrontal cortex (involved in the valuation of stimuli) and the hippocampus (involved with memory) work in conjunction to produce self-referential thought. The DMN has been called the "narrative network" (Bressler & Menon, 2010) because it provides the stream of self-referential internal dialogue that characterizes thoughts when people are not occupied. These thoughts tend to be self-focused and often self-critical.

On the other hand, functioning of the DEN is characterized by activity in the insula, which processes incoming sensory information, and the anterior cingulate cortex, which is involved with the attention mechanisms. Studies have demonstrated that when either the DEM or DMN is operational, the other is silent. Therefore, when people are involved with rich, sensory experiences, the DEN overrides the DMN and the narrative network is quiet. I hope that readers will try the sensory experiences described below and enjoy the experience of sensation itself, without the usual mental narrative in operation. The inner narrative is silenced when the experience does not have a goal. When there is an objective in mind, it is typical that the narrative becomes strong; the "internal critic" seems to continually evaluate the process and product. Total immersion in a sensory experience is one way to tame this inner critical voice. Grounding oneself in sensation is one way to increase mindfulness in the present, reducing sadness about the past or anxiety about the future. Pay attention to any one of the five senses to bring awareness back to the present time and experience a moment of relaxation.

Maximizing Sensual Pleasure

By its very nature, sensual pleasure is fleeting and short-lived. Sensations are signals, and as such they typically come and go rather quickly. However, there are proven ways to maximize engagement with and enjoyment of sensual pleasure, and therefore ensure that the sensations are as enriching as possible. First, it is important to be alert to sensual possibilities. This will require a slower pace of life so that attention can be devoted to sensual pleasures. Slowing down the pace of life also allows for engagement in the next technique for enhancing sensual pleasure, which is "savoring" (Hurley & Kwon, 2010). Savoring means that people spend at least 30 seconds immersed in a sensual experience: gazing or inhaling, swathed in touch or sound. Research supports that sensual pleasure and the resulting effects on mood are significantly increased by savoring sensations and experiences (Gentzler, Palmer, & Ramsey, 2016; Hurley & Kwon, 2012; Jose, Lim, & Bryant, 2012). Further, older adults who are better at savoring the positive aspects of life are significantly more satisfied with their lives than those who are not, regardless of their physical health status (Smith & Bryant, 2016).

The "First Time–Last Time" experience also helps intensify sensation. This means that when faced with a lovely sensation, people think, "what if this was the first time I ever saw, tasted, felt, etc. this particular thing?" Or "what if this were the last time I was ever to experience such a sensation?" This reverent attitude towards sensation can significantly magnify its experience. In addition, engaging in the first time–last time experience might increase overall appreciation and gratitude. Some believe that in our safe and healthy Western society we have lost vitality in our lives because we do not often face our deaths, or any "last time" experiences. During the Renaissance, it was common for people to have a human skull on their desk as a *memento mort*, a reminder that life was short and death was eminent. This memento was intended to encourage people to remain humble and to live their lives in ways that were pleasing to God.

Another way to enhance sensory enrichment is to avoid repetition of the same stimulus. Due to a phenomenon called habituation, any repeated sensation loses its excitatory ability – it is adaptive to habituate to familiar sensations because it allows those things that are different to stand out from the background of ordinary stimulation and signal potential threat or opportunity. For example, people notice that when they live with a painting for a long time, they no longer "see" it. However, when a new person enters the house and notices it, the painting is new again. It is also possible to encounter a familiar sensation so often that it becomes annoying. I worked with a client who was trying to break the habit of drinking coffee and decided to replace it with peach tea. She thought it would be a tasty and satisfying replacement for her beloved coffee; and it was enjoyable – for a while. Because peach tea was the only hot beverage she drank for a month, at the end of that time, she hated it. If she had varied the flavor of herbal tea she might not have liked them all, but she probably would not have hated the peach flavor. Therefore, the lesson is twofold – first, avoid repetition of sensory stimulation in order to reduce habituation and second, have a variety of self-care "flavors" or strategies in your arsenal so that one does not become noxious after a while. Variety is the spice of (an enriched) life.

Finally, sharing sensory stimulation with loved ones enhances its positive effects (Ferrucci, 2009; Hurley & Kwon, 2012). Sharing anything beautiful with loved ones is part of the work of love that strengthens connections and deepens bonds. Before the days of Facebook and Instagram, I asked my children to share with me a picture of something that they experienced as beautiful. Often a picture of something inspiringly beautiful arrives unexpectedly and without words; I know that they are saying, "I love you." Further, appreciating beauty in the natural world strengthens and deepens our connection with the divine. Barbara Brown Taylor writes in her book, *An Altar in the World* (2009), that it is nearly impossible to engage in the restful pleasures of admiring beauty because it is "revolutionary" to do so in our fast paced, product-oriented world. By taking the time to rest and enjoy without producing a product, we are going against the way that our society assigns value to people and experiences. Because it is difficult to be a lone revolutionary, she suggests finding a person or a community of other people who share the same values and who will support a practice of appreciation.

Summary and Conclusions

Sensory experiences can arouse awe, joy, and love, which all have significant positive effects on psychological, emotional, and physical health. Thus, sensory experiences inspire a significant portion of the deep well of positive emotion, compassion, and optimism that characterizes an enriched life. The wonderful thing about sensation is that people have five channels, available every moment of every day, through which to enrich their lives. Slowing down the pace of life increases opportunities for life enrichment because at a slower pace, people are better able to notice the beautiful sights around them, luxuriate in the sensual aspects of touch, and savor sumptuous tastes and aromas. A slower pace of life is conducive to appreciating silence, as well as mindfully adding enjoyable sounds such as favorite music.

Sensory enrichment grounds people in the present and reduces the probability that they experience sadness about the past or anxiety about the future. When people are fully present in the moment, their mindful presence slows down the perception of time, which helps establish the wide margins that are a hallmark of the enriched life. Living life with wide margins will increase the possibility of having, noticing, and immersing oneself in beauty. This growth of this virtuous cycle will counteract the "revolutionary" aspects of embracing beauty; more time is available to rest in sensuality with no pressure to produce anything.

The enrichment experienced through sensation can be heightened and prolonged. The pleasure derived from sensual experience is enhanced when people pay attention and spend at least 30 seconds savoring the moment, act as if this were the first time or last time they might experience the sensation, and avoid doing the same thing repeatedly. Finally, in order to enrich your life with sensation of any kind, it is important to mix it up. Vary the fantastic food that you eat. Try changing the scents that surround you once a week, or the familiar sights once a month. When the sensations you experience are many and varied, you will find greater joy in sensory stimulation.

Sensory Actions and Art Reflections

1. Go to one of your favorite places in nature and use the natural materials that you find there (rocks, sand, leaves, bark, and shells) to create a work of art or use the textures that you find to create a rubbing.
2. Use finger paints and finger paint paper and use the rich paint and smooth paper to experience the visual/tactile nature of these materials. Do not attempt to create anything in particular, but just notice the sensations of the paint gliding around the paper and the colors mixing.
3. Use traditional yarn, thread, cloth, or beads to make something that is an expression of an inner sensation. You do not have to create anything in particular; just notice the sensations of working with textiles and crafts. Notice if and how the experience of the inner sensation began to match outer sensation of the craftwork.
4. Find a unique way of sharing beauty with a special person in your life.

Questions for Self-Reflection

1. What did you notice in your body when you immersed yourself in sensual experiences? Were you feeling any emotion as you encountered these materials?
2. How did being involved with sensation (without regard to producing a final artistic product) influence the inner critical voice?

Life Enrichment through Movement 5

> *Me thinks that the moment my legs begin to move
> my thoughts begin to flow.*
> Henry David Thoreau (2009, p. 68)

Sensation is opposite from movement on the Life Enrichment Model, but both aspects are essential components of a healthy, enriched life. As was discussed in Chapter 3, there is a robust interplay between these two physical qualities of life – as involvement with one component goes up, the other goes down. This relationship between the two opposing sides of the model on this level means that as people become increasingly active, their ability to notice fine variations in sensation decreases. Eventually, vigorous exercise interferes with or overrides the ability to perceive fine variations in sensation, which can lead to an overall reduction in well-being if people do not listen to their bodies. Achieving a dynamic balance between sensory and movement experiences can decrease the possibility of injury and increase the likelihood of appropriate self-care. For example, after a run, if people pay attention to the physical sensations in the body, they will notice a need for rest and recuperation. They will likely balance the overload of physical activity with a sensory sensation like taking a relaxing, warm shower.

There has been a great deal of research demonstrating the myriad benefits of engaging in regular physical exercise above and beyond physical activity.

It is important to note that while physical activity and physical exercise are both important to well-being, they are two distinctly different entities. Physical activity usually refers to any sort of movement that involves the musculoskeletal system, whereas physical exercise is planned and repetitive activity done for the purpose of increasing physical fitness (Caspersen, Powell, & Christenson, 1985). When I write about the many benefits listed below, I am referring to the benefits of both regular physical exercise and physical activity; when the distinction is important I will make it. It is important to keep in mind that long periods of exercise are not necessary to feel its positive effects. An exercise physiologist that I worked with once said, "you don't have to get all of your exercise in one long sweaty session." Small amounts of activity can be effective. One study demonstrated that a physically active lunch break and a habit of taking the stairs rather than the elevator were both associated with lower self-rated "need for recovery" scores, meaning that people did not feel such a great need to rest after work when they were more consciously active during the day (Coffeng, van Sluijs, Hendriksen, van Mechelen, & Boot, 2015).

Benefits of Exercise

It is interesting to note that people who spend more of their leisure time in physical activity are more likely to rate themselves as optimally healthy (Galán, Meseguer, Herruzo, & Rodríguez-Artalejo, 2010). Regular physical exercise is associated with abundant life-enriching effects in both physical and psychological arenas (Ratey & Hagerman, 2008). In fact, there are so many positive benefits linked with regular physical exercise that it has been called the "self-control miracle" by health psychologists (McGonigal, 2013). This means that people who engage in regular physical exercise notice the positive effects and are therefore more likely to engage in other health-promoting habits such as eating nourishing foods, drinking plenty of water, avoiding addictive substances, and developing regular sleeping routines.

Engaging in physical activity frequently is associated not only with movement, but also with enjoying the outdoors. Therefore, the positive effects of movement are those that also are associated with encounters that simultaneously excite the senses and induce relaxation (Ratey & Manning, 2015). As was mentioned earlier, being in nature is associated with decreases in both objectively and subjectively rated measures of stress.

Increased Positive Emotions

Across all age groups, people who engage in regular workouts are more likely to experience increased positive emotions, feelings of subjective well-being, and improved self-image (Garcia, Archer, Moradi, & Andersson-Arntén, 2012; Kohn, Belza, Petrescu-Prahova, & Miyawaki, 2016). Perhaps by providing a container and outlet for stress, physical exercise and subsequent physical fitness can mitigate the stressful effects of a demanding occupation and reduce the likelihood of burnout (Schmidt, Beck, Rivkin, & Diestel, 2016). Kohn, et al. (2016) identified many additional psychosocial resources that are enhanced by physical exercise, including greater self-acceptance, increased sense of purpose and mastery, positive relationships, and social integration. Yoga is one type of physical exercise that has been shown to reduce stress by increasing positive emotions and self-compassion (Riley & Park, 2015).

In addition, many studies show that regular physical exercise has potent antidepressant effects for mild to moderate depression, especially for women (Zhang & Yen, 2015). Aerobic exercise has been used successfully in the treatment of various anxiety disorders (Powers, Asmundson, & Smits, 2015). Exercise seems to have longer-lasting effects than medication for people experiencing symptoms of mild to moderate depression. Researchers believe this is because exercise not only alters brain chemistry, but through increasing self-confidence and positive feelings towards the self, it changes one's whole sense of identity. The benefits of physical exercise are the greatest when the activity is perceived as pleasant. Pickett, Kendrick, & Yardley (2017) found that when exercise was enjoyable, rather than something merely accomplished, participants reported feeling more generally engaged in life. Further, they rated themselves as experiencing more positive emotions and the impetus for exercising changed from external (knowing exercise is good for them) to internal (wanting to exercise because it feels good). Internal or intrinsic motivation is more likely than external motivation to sustain a habit in the long term. So, to reduce the stress of a demanding and sedentary job as a therapist, make sure to include convenient and enjoyable exercise in your life.

Using art materials with movement can be a fun way to increase positive emotions and reduce stress. Plates 2 and 3 show two images created by people who, working outside, threw paint onto large pieces of paper without expectations of the final product. Although there was some initial fear of splashing paint on clothing, most described the experiences as: fun, invigorating, and "releasing". Art experience through movement can promote the physical and emotional release of energy and tension and reduce stress.

Improved Cognitive Functioning

Exercise improves a variety of different cognitive functions including attention, academic performance, and memory (Ratey & Hagerman, 2008). A ten-minute walk will return the brain to its most alert and the body to its most relaxed state of the day. This kind of activity break is often just what people need when their jobs require a great deal of sitting. Also, during a stressful time at home or work, taking a break for physical exercise is a great way to express the activation and work out the frustration (Sharma, Madaan, & Petty, 2006).

Helping Professionals take note: The next time you find yourself holding your breath and tensing your muscles with stress, take a brisk, 10-minute walk and allow this natural stress reliever to work for you. You will come back to your work with renewed attention and relaxed energy.

Hogan, Mata & Carstensen (2013) demonstrated that across all age groups, physical exercise improves working memory functioning. Improvements in attention seem to follow an inverted U-shaped model, with optimal improvement at moderate levels of exercise (Hüttermann & Memmert, 2012). Physical exercise has been shown to increase the number of neuronal connections in the brain and enhance all executive functioning. Exercise can make you smarter!

Enhanced Sleep

Regular physical exercise improves the overall quality of sleep in people across ages and life circumstances (Connaughton, Patman, & Pardoe, 2014; Flausino, Da Silva Prado, De Queiroz, Tufik, & De Mello, 2012; Hartescu, Morgan, & Stevinson, 2015; Kredlow, Capozzoli, Hearon, Calkins, & Otto, 2015). In addition, evidence shows that when people are well rested and physically fit, they are more able to meet the stressors that will inevitably enter their lives. I like to call this approach to stress "inoculation," meaning that one can build up resistance to stressors by being as healthy as possible in body, mind, and spirit. Exercise at any time during the day will improve sleep quality. However, the best time for exercise to improve sleep is not right before bedtime, but three to four hours prior. Exercise is associated with a rise in body temperature and a consequent drop in body temperature below baseline three to four hours later. This drop in body temperature allows for better sleep quality during the night (Breus, 2006).

Increased Strength

Aside from regular aerobic exercise, enriching life through movement can mean taking pleasure in one's strength and muscular ability, flexibility, agility, and motion. Enrichment through movement and the body means paying attention and honoring what your body can do rather than focusing on how your body looks. People who focus on what their bodies can do are less likely to develop disordered eating than those who maintain a vigilant stance on how their bodies look (Elavsky, 2010). Strengthening the body and taking pride in gaining fitness can occur through participating in training "boot camps," taking a martial arts class, going to the gym, engaging a personal trainer, or doing simple strength training exercises on your own.

When people take pleasure in what their bodies can do, they feel strong and well and their lives are physically enriched. For people whose mobility is challenged due to pain, disability, or other limitations, it is best to begin any exercise program with an evaluation by a physician, physical therapist, or exercise physiologist. Working together, these professionals can help determine individual strengths and weaknesses and help people determine when pain means harm and when to push through. Working with a professional can help people monitor and take pride in physical progress, while perhaps adding joy to physical activity where previously they might have felt frustration.

Decreased Fatigue

An ironic fact about general fatigue is that it is best combated with exercise which, if people are experiencing fatigue, they usually do not feel like doing. But it is true that for general fatigue (not necessarily the fatigue that results from illness), exercise is the antidote. The best type of exercise to decrease fatigue is a moderately intense 10–15-minute walk. This type of exercise generates "calm energy" and is characterized by a combination of high levels of physical and mental energy with low physical tension (Thayer, 2001). The opposite of calm energy is "tense energy," a static physical state distinguished by a high level of tension, which encourages the fast action and efficient task completion typical of Type A behavior. However, tense energy often degenerates into tense tiredness producing the general fatigue that many people complain about to their general practitioners (Thayer, 2001).

Physical activity can be a remedy for fatigue, but only if it does not become another source of stress (Strahler, et al., 2016). Therefore, it is important for

Helping Professionals to monitor stress levels and use exercise under moderate to low chronic stress conditions and use rest under high chronic stress conditions. Remember that there is a dynamic interplay between the two components of this level and every level of the LEM: Movement and sensation operate in opposite ways but both are physically enriching. Listen to your body to recognize when you need more exercise and when you need to use sensation to create relaxation and rest. You can increase "calm energy" by scheduling 10–15-minute walking breaks into your calendar. Setting electronic reminders will significantly increasing the likelihood that the exercise takes place.

Rhythmic Movement

Rhythmic movements of all types can help reduce tension, stress, and anxiety (Kinsbourne, 2011; Thayer, 2001). Studies show that chewing and grooming behaviors appear in rats that are under stress; engaging in these behaviors appears to help calm them. Stress activates dopamine circuitry in the limbic system of the brain, and with too much stress the basal ganglia take control of behavior over higher cortical systems, generating simple and instinctive rather than learned actions. Familiar repetitive movements moderate the dopamine effect and reduce arousal levels (Kinsbourne, 2011). Rhythmic movement also activates the cerebellum and releases norepinephrine in the locus coeruleus (LC), providing a calming effect. The LC is a brain structure located in the brainstem which plays a role in attention/arousal; people with AD/HD often use repetitive movements to increase task attention. In addition, the LC also is connected to the limbic system through the amygdala and plays a role in emotion regulation. Many people regulate tension or anxiety with repetitive or rhythmic motions such as nail biting, but because they cannot perceive that they can control these habits, they often do not feel good about them. However, a similar soothing rhythm is created when people knit, crochet, or engage in various other types of craftwork, and there is evidence that this soothing rhythm is one of the many characteristics of working with textiles that makes them so appealing and therapeutic (Collier, 2011).

The rhythmic squeezing of a soft ball has been shown to decrease stress, probably due to the alternating increase in tension and progressive relaxation that occurs through the motion. Commercial "stress balls," clay, or thinking putty™ are available for quick stress relief during the day. There are additional benefits to using a stress ball on cognition: Kim (2015) studied the difference between squeezing a soft ball or a hard ball on two types of creative thinking. The researcher found that squeezing a soft ball enhanced divergent thinking. In other words, squeezing a soft ball helped participants come up with a greater number of diverse answers to a question. Alternatively, squeezing a hard ball increased convergent thinking by allowing participants to settle on one answer to a problem.

Helping Professionals take note: Squeezing a stress ball, playing with clay during short breaks throughout the day, or crocheting in the evenings or on weekends – these are all rhythmic means of reducing stress and enriching the physical aspects of life.

Sharing Movement

If you would like to add an exercise program to your life or make your existing one more regular, do not think that you have to do it alone. Research shows that people are more likely to show up for exercise when someone is waiting for them. Having someone engage in physical activity with you may increase your feelings of self-efficacy or self-esteem, or it may just enable you do to it when you do not feel motivated (Plante, Gustafson, Brecht, Imberi, & Sanchez, 2011). Sharing movement might be through dance: dance classes, ballroom dancing, therapeutic movement or improvisational dancing. There are many studies that show dancing increases cognitive functioning, well-being, and quality of life (Koch, Kunz, Lykou, & Cruz, 2014; Quiroga Murcia, Kreutz, Clift, & Bongard, 2010; Rehfeld, et al., 2017). A recent study by Rehfeld and colleagues compared the effects of an 18-month dancing program to a traditional fitness-training program on balance and brain volume. After the programs both groups showed some increases in hippocampal volume – a brain area associated with memory functioning. However, the dancing group showed greater increases in this measure than the fitness-training group, along with greater improvements in balance scores. The researchers recommended dancing over traditional fitness programs because dancing not only involves aerobic fitness, but also sensorimotor stimulation. Dancing is cognitively demanding but enjoyable; people are more likely to participate in exercise when they are having fun.

Time is a significant limiting factor in life; people are so busy that they do not have enough time to do all of the things that they want to do. Therefore, if people can schedule exercise with a friend or family member with whom they want to spend time, they receive two benefits from the same activity. With no more time spent, they attain two important results: a physical one and a social one. On the other hand, if they have very little time for meditation, time alone with a walking meditation can be a way to improve emotional expressiveness (Kim & Ki, 2014) and use limited resources wisely. So, increase the power of movement in your life by getting active with the people you love.

Summary and Conclusions

Being physically active is a powerful part of living an enriched life. Regular physical exercise is one way to release the stress that builds up during the day in an emotionally demanding job. It has been called "the self-control miracle" because engaging in regular physical exercise increases the likelihood that people will engage in other health-enhancing behaviors such as eating nutritious food and maintaining a healthy weight. People have limited time and resources, so they are more likely to do something when they realize that it involves more than one associated benefit. Engaging in regular physical exercise not only reduces stress, but it also helps maintain an appropriate weight, improves sleep, increases relaxation and alertness, and enhances cognitive functioning and mood. Exercising with a friend provides additional motivation to continue the regimen (Scarapicchia, Amireault, Faulkner, & Sabiston, 2017), reduces the perception of difficulty, and allows people to do more with less perceived effort. Movement of any kind, but especially the repetitive movement involved in crocheting, knitting, or other crafts is a significant outlet for stress. Using art with vigorous movement can be a pleasurable way to reduce stress.

Across all ages, people who exercise regularly are likely to rate themselves as optimally healthy and to have greater energy and enjoyment of life. Because of its many health-promoting effects, regular physical exercise can be a tool for stress inoculation – it can increase strength, energy, and vitality while at the same time reducing stress, anxiety, and depression. Movement is one of the basic elements that create a deep reservoir of well-being characteristic of the enriched life and the excellent helping professional. Therapists who engage in regular exercise are inoculated against the effects of stress that inevitably will enter their lives as they counsel those who seek their help.

Movement and Art Reflections

1. Work with natural clay – kneading, rolling, and moving with the resistive yet flexible material without thinking that you have to create anything in particular.
2. Working outside, create an image by throwing liquid paint onto a large paper or canvas set upon the ground.
3. Make sure that you find a way of sharing movement with someone you love; dance in a way that is meaningful, go for a bike ride together, or take a hike in beautiful, natural surroundings.

Questions for Self-Reflection

1. How did your body feel before, during, and after one of the movement exercises? Did you notice a feeling of relaxation occurring after the activity?
2. What sort of regular physical exercise are you willing to commit to as a way to enrich your life?
3. What friend or family member can you include in your new systematic plan for exercise? How will they provide additional inspiration or motivation? How will you motivate them?

Life Enrichment through Pattern and Routine   6

> *Perhaps there is a pattern set up in the heavens for one who desires to see it, and having seen it, to find one in himself.*
>
> Plato (1945, p. 319)

Moving up the Life Enrichment Model, we come to the middle level, which focuses on pattern and routine on one side, and emotion on the other. As was mentioned in a previous chapter, because there is an inverse relationship between the two components on each level, getting involved with action on one side will reduce activity on the other. Therefore, the relationship between the two components on the middle level of the model demonstrates that familiar patterns and routines can calm, ease, or comfort emotions like anxiety or anger. Furthermore, a dynamic balance between the two components is best so that routine does not become boring but is enlivened by emotion. Research on successful health care professionals describes how experts use physical, mental or spiritual routines to decompress and transition from working life to home life at the end of a day (Figley & Ludick, 2017; Harrison & Westwood, 2009).

Helping Professionals take note: Develop a mental routine in which you use your daily commute home from work to intentionally clear your mind and decompress from the workday. Adding your favorite musical theme song would be appropriate on particularly stressful days. A daily walk after work can afford a physical and/or spiritual cleansing from the cares of the day.

This chapter will explore patterns of viewing and acting in the world and how attention to these patterns and routines can enrich life. In particular, it will describe how a focus on pattern or routine can be a container for difficult emotions. Joyce Carol Oates, in an interview regarding the publication of her memoir *A Widow's Story*, demonstrated this concept when she pointed out that routine can promote creativity and enrich life. She stated,

> The domestic lives we live – which may be accidental, or not entirely of our making – help to make possible our writing lives; our imaginations are freed, or stimulated by the very prospect of companionship, quiet, a predictable and consoling routine.
> (Joyce Carol Oats Writes Memoir of Grief, 2011)

This chapter also will explore the principle of isomorphism and how it explains the reciprocal relationship between the external world and our internal experience of it. Finally, this chapter will address the development and cultivation of relational diversity to improve relationships; it examines the use of mandalas to reduce stress and increase calm and other uses of line, pattern and form for life enrichment.

The Comfort of Routines and Patterns

It is important to note that life enrichment does not require that people regularly add new activities to their lives. Remember that I wrote in the first chapter that I did not want this book to prompt the creation of a "to do list." People already engage in many life-enriching endeavors, and continuing to do them with greater mindful attention will increase their power. Life can be enriched by what is usual and customary. The repetition of well-learned patterns and routines in life offers comfort in familiarity: Notice how infants and children respond to the similarity of morning or evening routines. When they were young, my children came to expect that stories would follow baths and lead to bed. The routine soothed them to sleep. For children, when all is carried out in a predictable order behavior is calm; a break in routine is unsettling (causes negative emotions) and provokes disruptive behavior. Adults are similarly soothed by familiar routines in their lives (Duhigg, 2014). Thomas Merton emphasized this point in writing about happiness, "Happiness is not a matter of intensity but of balance and order and rhythm and harmony" (Merton, 1983, p. 127).

Routines, when not too rigid, provide a structure to life that allows people to relax into their days without putting conscious thought into every action or decision. Imagine the energy that it would take to consciously think through each behavior (from tooth brushing in the morning to putting the dishes in the dishwasher after dinner) – routines save time and energy. They allow more time for the things that people want to do by organizing the activities that they have to do. Routines also aid new habit formation because it is easier to attach a new behavior to an existing one. People who have strong habitual patterns in their lives can add new links with less effort than it would take to begin a completely new routine (Duhigg, 2014). A bedtime routine can improve sleep because of the regulation of the internal clock by the familiarity of nighttime activities performed at similar times each evening (Breus, 2006).

Isomorphism

Isomorphism is a principle taken from mathematics, which literally means equal (iso) shape (morph). In math, two structural models demonstrate isomorphism when all of the elements correspond with one another (Arnheim, 1966). In art therapy, the term isomorphism has been used to explain that people project onto art materials and process and portray in their art products what they are thinking and feeling; art is seen as a mirror of the artist's interior life. In Gestalt psychology, isomorphism explains how physiological processes in our bodies respond to physical processes and structures in our world (Arnheim, 1966). Because of the physiological processes operating within us (including the work of mirror neurons) during our responses to our environment, we can take on the feeling of our surroundings. This means that in contemplating life enrichment, it is essential to be aware of design elements in the environment. The physical environment can enrich or detract from the quality of life. If a person's surroundings are cluttered or messy, they will tend to feel uneasy, restless, or stressed. If the environment is neat and organized, people will take on the feeling of those surroundings and feel calm. Therefore, organizing closets and drawers and de-cluttering spaces and surfaces can be a relatively easy way to improve the quality of your life.

Apparently, there is a great need for information about clearing out closets and cupboards. Author Marie Kondo published *The Life-Changing Magic of Tidying Up* in October 2014, and 14 months later it became a #1 *New York Times* bestseller. Two years later, the book had been on the bestseller list for 100 weeks. Clearly, many people want to feel better about how their possessions are taking over their surroundings, but need help with downsizing and de-cluttering. To reduce procrastination and begin the process of tidying up, it can be helpful to read a book about how to start the organizing project. Even more useful might be to have a friend help or to call a professional organizer. Having an objective person involved in the process can help people stay on task with the sorting, storing, and tossing of things that are no longer useful or meaningful.

Mandala Coloring

Long before the current coloring book craze, there were mandala coloring books based on the work of psychoanalyst Carl Jung and art therapist Joan Kellogg (Fincher, 2000). Mandala comes from a Sanskrit word meaning "sacred circle" and it is believed that creating in this archetypal form is centering and healing. Mandala coloring can take the form of filling in a small, prepared circular design such as the one in Plate 4, or creating a free form design with the template of a plate-sized circle. Completing the circle in the first chapter of this book was an exercise in mandala coloring. Creating in the form of a circle is believed to contain troubling emotion, putting boundaries around the emotion so that it can be experienced as non-threatening or so that the impact of the emotion can be reduced to a manageable level. To support this hypothesis, many studies have demonstrated that drawing or painting in the sacred circle of a mandala can reduce subjective ratings of stress and anxiety and decrease negative mood (Babouchkina & Robbins, 2015; Curry & Kasser, 2005; Henderson, Rosen, & Mascaro, 2007; Kersten & van der Vennet, 2010; van der Vennet & Serice, 2012). Researchers have refined their studies to specify that it is the circular form that contains emotion, not another geometric shape (Babouchkina & Robbins, 2015).

Lines Can Aid Meditation

Aside from reducing stress and repairing negative mood, the use of pattern and form can aid meditation. Lines drawn, one after another in a repetitive fashion, can help focus attention in the present moment, perhaps in the same way that a Buddhist monk might experience a mindful moment while raking the small stones of a Zen garden into repetitious, wave-like patterns. One method of using lines in this repetitive fashion is Zentangle™ (Hall, 2012).

Life Enrichment through Pattern & Routine 53

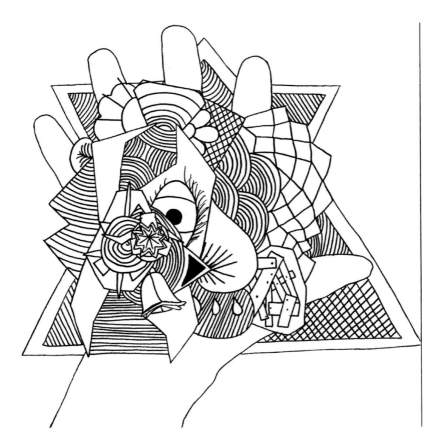

Figure 6.1 Zentangle: Lines Aid Meditation

The basic Zentangle™ begins with making a small scribble with a light pencil stroke in a small, four-inch square. The size restriction of the Zentangle™ is one element of the drawing that keeps it manageable and meditative. In the next step, various types of lines are added in the spaces where the lines of the original scribble intersected one another. Lines can be straight or curved, horizontal or vertical, plain or highly decorative. As can be seen in the drawing presented in Figure 6.1, the process is unlimited. One suggestion, however, is that the drawings not be intended to represent a particular object, because focusing on a specific shape can reduce the meditative quality of the drawing experience. Books and classes on the Zentangle™ process can help increase the enjoyment and benefits received through the practice.

Following on the heels of Zentangle™ there has been a spate of coloring books targeted at adult audiences. These coloring books have much more intricate designs than those made for children, and adults are free to use markers or colored pencils to complete their drawings rather than standard children's crayons. Coloring books are touted as stress relieving, meditative, mindful, calming therapy, color therapy, creative therapy, and art therapy. The coloring books clearly do not represent professional art therapy: The technique is not administered by a registered art therapist in controlled therapeutic conditions. However, it is likely that some of these activity books can be therapeutic, similar to the other ways of using lines and patterns as part of a meditative practice presented in this chapter. Becoming occupied with the ever-evolving designs can be a way to focus attention, or distract from other cares and concerns. Distraction is commonly cited as one therapeutic mechanism behind coloring (Forkosh & Drake, 2017) and is taught as an essential emotional regulation strategy (Liu & Thompson, 2017).

Doodling is another type of drawing activity that recently has received a great deal of media attention for its beneficial effects. Again, doodling is not a specific form of art therapy, but does focus on the use of art for therapeutic benefit. Doodling can have positive effects on cognitive processes such as attention and memory (Andrade, 2010; Brown, 2015; Singh, & Kashyap, 2015). It has been shown that doodling while listening to a person speaking significantly boosts subsequent memory retrieval (Andrade, 2010; Singh & Kashyap, 2015). In her class on the workings of the mind, professor Lynda Barry requires her students to create doodles as they listen to lectures in order to enhance their attention to and retention of the course material (Barry, 2014). Observational data supports the role of doodling in stress reduction, possibly because this unfocused drawing activity distracts the default mode network of the brain (Schott, 2011). As was mentioned in the last chapter, the default mode network is that part of the brain that is working when people are not actively engaged in a task. It is operational when they are not busy and when not busy, people tend to worry. Doodling is an easy but engaging task that can reduce worry and increase attention.

Sharing Pattern and Perception

Representational Diversity

Typical ways of perceiving the world provide us with reassurance, but no one wants to become so inured in the way that they see things that they cannot change, or so rigid that they insist that their way of viewing a situation is the only correct one. Always having to be right is a cognitive distortion or an inaccurate way of thinking that amplifies negative emotions (Burns, 2008; De Oliveira, et al., 2015). People who always want to be right also tend to come across as righteous and offensive to others. Exploring and cultivating new ways of perceiving the world enriches lives and can aid the survival of our relationships. If life enrichment is to be sustained over time, a flexible, dynamic balance among experiences and ways of perceiving is required, including the ability to perceive things from another person's perspective.

The term representational diversity refers to the ability to see things from another person's point of view (Hinz, 2009). Being able to see things from a loved one's perspective enriches the relationship. When this cognitive understanding is combined with emotional understanding, the term "empathic accuracy" is used. Empathic accuracy refers to how accurately a person can infer the feelings and thoughts of another (Sened, et al, 2017). Research demonstrates that empathic accuracy grows over the course of committed, long-term relationships. When people demonstrate increasing empathic accuracy in perceiving their partner, a deep sense of being known and understood develops that is correlated with increased relationship satisfaction (Sened, et al., 2017). For those of us in the helping professions, it is also important to cultivate empathic accuracy with clients. The term "exquisite empathy" has been used to describe the way in which expert practitioners engage their clients with deep empathic accuracy, but with firm boundaries. Preserving clear boundaries allows us to express empathy and encourage work within the therapeutic bond without confusing client emotional expression with our own (Harrison & Westwood, 2009).

Patterns, shapes, and lines can be the rudimentary tools for improving empathic accuracy and relational diversity, while also enhancing relationships. For instance, looking at optical illusions – pictures that can be seen in two ways – can allow informal but significant exploration of relational diversity. Take for example Figure 6.2, which depending on how it is viewed, can be seen as either a beautiful young woman or an ugly old witch. Conversation on neutral or positive topics such as optical illusions can encourage alternative perspective taking as an exercise in increasing relational diversity.

In addition, the longer people look at something (prolonged inspection), the more likely they are to notice and appreciate its secondary characteristics, allowing them a diversity of perception that they would not have had if they only gave an object the usual, cursory glance (Arnheim, 1966). This too is sound advice in relationships – take adequate time to really look at a situation, a person, or a thing before reacting to it. Taking time for consideration can

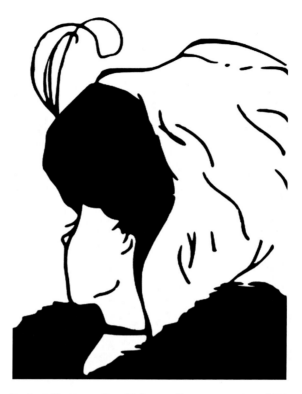

Figure 6.2 Optical Illusions Can Enhance Representational Diversity

lead to a proactive and rational response rather than a reactive and emotional response. As therapists we must allow ample time to consider the unique needs of the clients we are working with before making judgments about their behavior.

Being able to see things from a partner's perspective can reduce the likelihood that people labor under the belief that they have to be right or that they have to have the last word. I have noticed in my own life as a parent, for example, that if I raise my voice when disagreeing with my children, they will yell too. If I insist on getting the last word in an argument, then the last thing that my teenagers hear as they leave the room is my raised voice, allowing them to ruminate on what a lousy mother I am. If I raised my voice then I feel like a terrible mother and soon I am on my way to apologize for starting an argument and for saying things that I did not mean. Seeing things from another person's perspective reduces the likelihood that people cause or escalate an argument by having to have the last word.

Setting Boundaries

One function of lines is to define areas that create shapes, territories, and boundaries. This is a good metaphor for one of the important features of the successful Helping Professional: the ability to set firm boundaries around time spent at work so that time and resources are available for life enrichment and self-care (Harrison & Westwood, 2009). Setting good boundaries includes taking stock of personal strengths and limitations and creating a schedule that allows people to thrive in the setting(s) where they work. Early career professionals are particularly susceptible to saying yes to every opportunity that presents itself in order to create professional connections and future work opportunities. However, many often find that having agreed to many small commitments leaves them with too much time allotted for work each week and little or no time for leisure and enrichment.

It is important to believe that saying no to occasional requests and reserving time for oneself is not selfish; it is necessary self-preservation. Dr. Brené Brown, the author of *The Gifts of Imperfection* (2010), notes that compassionate people have definite boundaries. They do not say yes to every request of their time and talent. When people say no to some requests, they can say a more genuine and resounding yes to others. If people aid everyone who asks for their help, if they give in to those who make inappropriate requests, then they can wind up feeling resentful of everyone who asks for their help, even those to whom they legitimately want to give.

When people say yes to everything, requests start feeling like demands and instead of giving with grace, people can become burned out and give unwillingly. Family members, friends, and patients can notice when their requests are unwelcome (even when they are granted) and then they feel ashamed for having asked. No one ends up feeling good when boundaries are not firm. Compassionate support comes from an open and loving heart, not an angry one. When therapists set good limits on the amount of time and energy that they spend on others, they have more of those important resources available for other and for life enrichment (Harrison & Westwood, 2009). Therefore, it is important to remember that saying "no" is an integral part of self-preservation and being optimally healthy.

Boundaries are not permanent once settled upon; in fact over time they are very likely to require modification. As the demands of your life change – you get a pet, get married, have a child, or a parent requires care – the amount of time that you want to spend with family or at work will change. Therefore, it is important to assess regularly whether or not the important territories of life need new lines of demarcation. I suggest that people do some sort of self-reflective activity (in art, writing or both) at the beginning of each new year (calendar or academic) to evaluate the various aspects of their lives (occupational, social, familial, leisure, and spiritual) and whether they need to devote more or less time to any of them.

Summary and Conclusions

Life enrichment does not mean that people have to constantly look for new activities to add to their lives. The familiar patterns and routines in life bring people comfort. Flexible routines can provide a daily structure that allows people to relax and conserve energy because they do not have to think through every decision. They help us sleep better, get more done, and organize our environment to feel calm and relaxed. Routines also help us more easily form new habits, by allowing us to add one element to an existing solid pattern in our lives. Pattern and routine in art can aid relaxation or meditation by helping us focus on the present moment, providing containment or distraction from negative emotions. Sharing patterns and perceptions with loved ones can enrich people's lives by allowing them to appreciate their loved one's point of view, and this type of sharing not only enhances relationships but increases their durability and longevity.

Patterns and routines help therapists create and maintain good boundaries in their professional and personal relationships. Being a good therapist requires empathic accuracy; one has to be able to accurately perceive and appropriately respond to the feelings of another. The attention and devotion required to develop empathic accuracy requires psychic and physical energy. Firm boundaries help therapists ensure that their energy is dedicated to clients when appropriate and to self when applicable. With appropriate boundaries in place, the likelihood of therapists developing exquisite empathy increases and the chances of compassion fatigue or other harmful conditions resulting their work are reduced.

Pattern and Routine Art Reflection

1. On a 12″ × 18″ sheet of drawing paper, trace the outline of a dinner plate in pencil. Use a ruler to create a square inside the circle and then a triangle inside the square. Add any other geometric shape(s) that you want and then color in a pattern with markers, colored pencils or pastels.

2. On a small sheet of drawing paper (6" × 9") create a personal doodle by starting with a random shape or line and then adding repetitive lines and shapes.
3. On a small square piece of paper (4" × 4") create a quick scribble with a loose stroke. Make sure that some lines intersect. In the spaces created by the intersecting lines, add lines of any type (horizontal, vertical, curvilinear) in a repetitive fashion. Repeat with different strokes until all of the spaces are filled.
4. Trace a jar lid onto paper seven times. Create a small, free-form mandala drawing each day for a week (at the same time of day) to express your hopes for the day to come (morning mandala) or your feelings about the day that passed (evening mandala).

Questions for Self-Reflection

1. What bodily sensations did you notice as you were coloring the mandala you created? Were you immersed in the activity? Did a feeling of relaxation follow?
2. Try doodling as you listen to an instructive YouTube video or a 20-minute Ted Talk. What effect did the doodling have on your normal attention processes? How could doodling be incorporated into your day to enrich your listening experiences?
3. If you completed one small mandala per day, what did you notice about the experience that enriched your day?
4. Reflect on a physical, mental, or spiritual routine that you could implement to help you successfully transition from work to home each day. Could music, nature, or art comprise a meaningful part of that routine?

Life Enrichment through Emotion

7

> *There are moments in life, when the heart is so full of emotion*
> *That if by chance it be shaken, or into its depths like a pebble*
> *Drops some careless word, it overflows, and its secret,*
> *Spilt on the ground like water, can never be gathered together.*
> Henry Wadsworth Longfellow (1884, p. 212)

According to Swiss psychiatrist and psychoanalyst Carl Jung, "Emotion is the chief source of all becoming conscious. There can be no transforming of darkness into light and of apathy into movement without emotion" (Jacobi, 1961, p. 32). I believe that this quote aptly describes the necessity of emotion for transformation. Bestowing this significance on emotion is fitting, as emotions can be life-saving signals. This chapter will explore how various aspects of emotional experiences can not only be life saving, but life enriching as well. Enriching life with emotion does not just mean increasing the amount of positive emotion that we experience, but also befriending and embracing all emotions, seeing them as a major energizing and organizing life force. Emotions provide us with important information about needs and fuel our decision making. They help people set boundaries in their personal and professional lives. Finally, positive emotions build psychological resources that promote resilience in the excellent Helping Professional.

Chapter 3 explained that the second level of the Life Enrichment Model corresponds to activity in brain areas called the limbic system or the mammalian brain (Lusebrink, 2004; 2010; MacLean, 1985). The limbic structures of the brain give mammals and humans the ability to analyze well-known and unknown patterns in their surroundings and to respond with corresponding emotional signals. Pattern similarities confirm the status quo; similarities send a signal that the environment is as expected and no emotional alarm is generated. Patterns not seen before – discrepancies in design, line, shape, and color – elicit emotional signals because these differences represent opportunities or threats to survival. Moreover, if an animal or human breaks routine and behaves unexpectedly, members of the community are alerted or distressed by this change in expected or patterned behavior. The distress prompts new responses in the witness. Therefore, the limbic system functions as a moderator between urgent messages from the environment and action in the environment.

The Purpose of Emotions

Emotions have been demonstrated to be evolutionarily conserved, life-saving signals of threat or opportunity, "hard wired" into people of every culture, identifiable by specific facial expressions from infancy onwards (Ekman, 2007). Intriguing new research shows that learning, both personal and cultural, influences our perceptions of emotion much more that originally believed (Feldman Barrett, 2017). The fact that learning plays a role in the development of emotions means that we also have the capacity to learn how to respond differently in the presence of emotion. As was mentioned in Chapter 3, one aspect of living an enriched life is to learn to respond intentionally rather than automatically in response to emotional signals. And whether they are predominately innate or responsive to learning, each of the six primary emotions (anger, sadness, fear, happiness, interest/surprise, and disgust) functions as a protective signal (Ekman, 2007; Goleman, 2005).

The most commonly discussed example of an emotional signal is that of fear. Fear signals the presence of a threat in the environment. It signals the animal or person to fight, flee, freeze, or faint in order to save its life (Bracha, 2004; Ekman, 2007). The five other primary emotions function in a similar way – they indicate the presence of threat or opportunity and encourage action to safeguard life. Although the physical existence of most people in our Western society is not threatened on a daily basis, people still maintain the ability to analyze the patterns of the environment and send and receive emotional signals based on what they perceive. According to Seligman (2011), the modern day purpose of negative emotions is to warn us about danger, while the purpose of positive emotions is to build social and psychological capital, a storehouse of beneficial traits and states that can be called upon for strengthening self and relationships.

Increasing Positive Emotions

All human beings have an evolutionarily adaptive and culturally influenced negativity bias which causes them to put more weight on negative factors than positive ones (Rozin & Royzman, 2001; Seligman, 2011). The negativity bias is adaptive, because paying attention to what might hurt them can keep people out of harm's way. The downside of the negativity bias is that it can increase feelings of disappointment, despair, and depression. One aspect of life enrichment by emotion is to thoughtfully increase positive emotions such as joy, interest, pride, and love. Research has shown that these positive emotions can be enhanced through simple yet effective means (Seligman, 2011). Positive emotions enrich people's lives by broadening their ability to think of proactive solutions to problems, along with their ability to act upon these solutions by building social, intellectual, and physical resources (Fredrickson, 2001).

According to Martin Seligman's book *Flourish: A Visionary New Under-Standing of Happiness and Well-being*, one way to significantly increase positive emotions is through reflecting on and writing down "what went well today, and why." Focusing on what went well counters the inherent tendency to see the self, the world, and the future in a pessimistic light. When people change the focus of their attention to the positive, it is possible to construct an inner reality that is largely optimistic. This positive construction brought about by focusing on "what went well" has powerful and long-lasting antidepressant effects (Seligman, 2011).

Another way to increase positive emotions is to focus attention on gratitude (Lambert, Fincham, & Stillman, 2012; Hanson & Hanson, 2018). There has been an explosion of research on gratitude in the last few years, showing that recording feelings of gratitude increases not only positive emotions, but also long-lasting feelings of subjective well-being and indicators of physical health (Emmons & McCullough, 2003; Jackowska, Brown, Ronaldson, & Steptoe, 2016; Lambert, et al., 2012; Nezlek, Newman, & Thrash, 2017). The most common way to increase feelings of gratitude is to keep a gratitude journal. This can be in the form of a quick daily record (sketch or list) of that for which one is uniquely thankful, a weekly journal entry in prose or poetry, or a gratitude visit. A gratitude visit entails writing a letter of appreciation to a person who had a significant positive impact on your life and making an appointment to read the letter to them in person (Seligman, 2011). All of these activities build resiliency, which allows people to broaden and build personal and positive resources that are life enriching.

Sharing Emotion

The experience of emotion in today's world is not usually life saving – though their lives are not threatened on a daily basis, people continue to experience emotions. The function of emotions today is not to save lives, but to save important relationships. Sharing activities merely draws people together; sharing emotions is what strengthens bonds and deepens relationships into intimacy. I can work with someone for years and not consider her a good friend because we have only shared the experience of working together. When I share my stresses, joys, or fears with my co-worker and my sharing is reciprocated, our relationship has the opportunity to develop into friendship. Further, if a person does not share emotions (either positive or negative) in the context of an important relationship, it is likely that the relationship will not grow closer or that the individuals will grow apart (L'Abate, 2016).

When Helping Professionals withhold rather than share important emotional reactions, especially negative emotions like fear, anger, and sadness, usually it is because the role of caretaker tacitly implies that these emotions should not be experienced. When therapists experience negative emotions about their work, the anticipated shame at being perceived as "weak" can preclude them from sharing them with others (Bilodeau, Savard, & Lecomte, 2012). In addition, therapists might have been raised in families or cultures where the darker emotions were not disclosed, and still are not shared as a habit learned long ago (Greenspan, 2003). Moreover, therapists usually are sensitive and perceptive; they can tell when their stories cause negative feelings in others and over time they can become reluctant to share the emotional aspects of their work. Therefore, they present a false self to others – one that they believe others want to encounter. But the false self is a lie, and in living this lie over time, their important relationships become shallow and unfulfilling. Whatever the reason for internalizing emotions, the habit can impede therapist effectiveness and harm personal mental and physical health (Hollis, 2008; Rogerson, Gottlieb, Handelsman, Knapp, & Younggren, 2011). Grief not expressed can become depression; fear kept inside can morph into prejudice and rage. Unexpressed despair can lead to a desire for numbing and addiction (Greenspan, 2003).

Across all studies of the effects of being a Helping Professional, supportive supervisory and social relationships are mentioned as significant elements of an enriched, life-enhancing practice (Figley & Ludick, 2017; Malinowski, 2014; McCormack & Adams, 2016; Newell, et al., 2016; Turgoose & Maddox, 2017; Železkov-Dorić, et al., 2012). Having a trusted mentor or peer with whom to share emotional reactions about professional work allows the distance necessary for the identification, understanding, expression, and resolution of troubling feelings. In the context of a supportive relationship, it is possible to discover the growth potential of the difficult emotions sometimes provoked by performing clinical work.

Emotion Regulation

Despite what a literal reading of the name might imply, emotion regulation does not just involve rules or guidelines for controlling emotions. Emotion regulation is a vast field of study which has to do with understanding the purpose of emotions, being able to access emotions when needed, identifying emotions as experienced, expressing and soothing emotions appropriately, and the complex relationships among all of these factors (Goleman, 2005; Gross, 2014; Lomas, Hefferon, & Ivtzan, 2014). Each aspect of emotion regulation can enhance professional abilities and personal relationships. Once therapists understand the purpose of emotions as signals, they can become more curious about what they feel in response to their clinical work and how those feelings were generated. This curiosity can fuel the necessary self-reflection required for being an excellent clinician. When the experience of emotion is conscious, therapists can be more aware of their needs and more confident in satisfying them.

One intention of work as a Helping Professional is to accompany clients on a journey into the unknown, into the pain of the past, holding space for the promise of a positive future. This deeply personal work evokes myriad emotions, and as we saw in the last chapter, patterns and routines can provide constructive ways of soothing the emotional reactions evoked in the course of working with people and their suffering. Helping Professionals can intentionally use physical, mental, or spiritual routines to decompress and transition home after work (Figley & Ludick, 2017; Harrison & Westwood, 2009). A planned transition from work will allow the clinician to leave work behind and successfully re-enter and re-engage with family members at the end of a stressful work day.

A former student of mine who worked as an art therapist in a pediatric hospital shared that she experienced secondary traumatic stress due to the emotionally draining therapy conducted with chronically ill children and their families (Gibson, 2017). She wanted to be present with her husband and three children, but frequently felt emotionally trapped at work, remembering the illnesses and deaths and re-experiencing her sadness. The therapist decided to use a visual journal as a way to transition from work to home. At the end of each work day, she took 30 minutes and created two pages (one in art and one in writing) in her journal. She used this routine as a container for her feelings so that they would remain at work and not leak over into her family life. She found that after a few weeks of using the visual journal she experienced significantly fewer symptoms of secondary traumatic stress and was more engaged with her family.

Helping Professionals take note: These are Diana Gibson's tips for successfully using a visual journal to contain emotions and transition from work to home without the emotional hangover: Keep your journal at work in a private, secure place. Inform colleagues that you will use some time at the end of your work day (after work but before going home) for art and writing and that you will likely not respond if interrupted. Ask their support in keeping your time private and uninterrupted. Create and write for 30 minutes, no exceptions (Gibson, 2017).

Emotional containment that occurs through visual journaling or other means can be beneficial and effective for reducing emotional distress, but in the extreme it can lead to compartmentalization or denial of painful emotions. Compartmentalization of emotions can reduce the likelihood of effective responding in difficult professional situations (Rogerson, et al., 2011). Therapists come into the practice of counseling for many different reasons, some of which are not conscious and may have to do with unmet personal needs, a desire to better understand themselves, or a need to work through their own problems (Kottler, 2017). When emotions are high, such as in challenging professional situations, unconscious needs and desires can influence behavior that may cause unintentional harm to clients. Difficult professional situations provoke thoughts that do not always follow rational and linear processes; these thoughts are unintentionally influenced by emotions, biases, and heuristics. Therefore, clinicians are likely to avoid errors in judgment when they take time to engage in self-reflective practices and understand their emotions and habitual inclinations before acting (Hollis, 2008).

Emotions and Decision Making

It is paramount that therapists are aware of judgments and resulting behavior that can be influenced by heuristics and biases. Heuristics and biases have been described as mental shortcuts and habitual ways of thinking that quickly, powerfully, and unconsciously influence decision making and problem solving (Rogerson, et al., 2011). Because they are customary ways of thinking, heuristics and biases often are not thought through before implementation; they are automatic. They allow for decision making that is efficient and rapid. Traditional beliefs are one type of heuristic that influences behavior. I have worked with nurses, therapists, and clergy who ascribed to what they described as traditional Christian beliefs, and within this belief system they characterized self-care as selfish. They consistently put other people's needs ahead of their own without thinking because "it is the Christian thing to do," but before long they were depleted and resentful. They eventually came to experience taking care of others as a duty, not as a delight. Another type of mental shortcut is the affect heuristic which, as the name implies, involves emotion. When the affect heuristic is at work, the strong emotion coloring a difficult situation quickly and powerfully influences a decision without conscious input. People rashly make decisions that will rapidly reduce their uncomfortable emotions, not understanding that it was discomfort rather than logic that motivated them (Rogerson, et al., 2011). Slowing down and reflecting in the presence of strong emotion can counteract the affect heuristic.

Self-reflection through creativity can allow for greater understanding of the emotional factors involved in clinical work. When therapists take time to identify their feelings, understand them, and express them in meaningful ways, their personal and professional lives are enriched. In response to emotions experienced during the course of the day, therapists can create images to contain and express those feelings. I created the images in Plate 5 and 6 in to express my emotions and thoughts in response to working with a depressed and suicidal client. The mixed media image in Plate 5 was created after a session in which the young man painted about and talked of his wishes and plans to die. My image of the crow as a harbinger of death helped me empathize with his sadness and self-destructive impulses. The ticket stub was added with its pleading message, "keep this coupon" as an expression of my desperate wish to keep him alive. The second image (Plate 6) was created in response to the first as a reparative (to me) expression of my hope for this young man. The crow also is celebrated for its intelligence and resiliency.

It is seen as a symbol of change, flexibility, and adaptability. My intention in creating this image was to reinforce that through our work together change could come about in a constructive way.

Furthermore, taking time to play a musical instrument or listen to music can be a way of managing the emotional tone of a difficult encounter. Ruud (2013) reported on the many ways that people deliberately engage with music to increase their well-being. The author called music a "cultural immunogen" for the effects that it has as a significant social and emotional resource and the way that it operates in emotion regulation.

Helping Professionals take note: Create playlists of songs for various emotional states and emotional needs. These can include songs that you know will cheer you up when you are sad, songs that will get you going when motivation is flagging, songs to match happy moods, and songs to channel anger in a productive way.

In addition to music, self-reflection also can be encouraged by mindfulness meditation, writing, engaging in supervision, talking with trusted peers or mentors, engaging in personal therapy, and viewing art. Viewing art is not a passive affair, but an active one that occurs as the viewer takes in what the artist intended and processes all types of information: visual, cognitive, emotional, and psychomotor (Chatterjee, 2015). Art can be a gentle way to invite emotion in: to explore, identify, share and express emotion. Each of the above mentioned activities can enrich your life as you embrace emotion as an important source of information. These creative emotional activities can increase energy rather than drain it.

Summary and Conclusions

Because emotions tend to build up when therapists accompany their clients through difficult life transitions, there are potential negative effects of not understanding and expressing emotion. However, the accumulation of emotion does not have to result in a harmful outcome for the practitioner. It is possible for Helping Professionals to develop resiliency skills in the context of arduous clinical work. Researchers have discovered that trauma counselors do not inevitably experience vicarious trauma, they can develop vicarious resilience. Vicarious resilience is a state characterized by a positive impact on the therapist's personal growth resulting from exposure to client resilience (Edelkott, Engstrom, Hernandez-Wolfe, & Gangsei, 2016). Elements of vicarious resilience include transformations in the therapist's self-perception and worldview, an enhanced sense of spirituality, a renewed commitment to self-care efforts, and a modified view of the therapeutic relationship. When therapists undergo vicarious resiliency, their new view of the therapeutic relationship is appreciably more strengths-based than deficit-focused. The relationship also is viewed as client-led rather than seen as the therapist being in charge. All of these elements coincide with an enriched and optimistic view of one's life work and purpose.

Enrichment through emotion means increasing positive emotions such as joy, interest, gratitude, and love. It also concerns tending to the darker emotions that are more difficult to understand and express. Identification of emotions, discrimination among them, understanding their functions, and learning accurate and healthy emotional expression are all part of living a life rich with emotion. Life enrichment through emotion involves embracing the energy that is provided by emotion and intentionally, rather than unconsciously, allowing emotion to influence decisions and behavior.

Research has demonstrated that in the face of the strong emotions evoked by performing clinical work, therapists often default to relying on unconscious cognitive shortcuts and biases when engaging in ethical decision making. Therefore, it is essential that therapists understand how to access their emotions and how to reflect on them to increase understanding, to communicate them if fitting, and to soothe them appropriately. Visual journaling was one technique suggested to help promote the identification, understanding, and expression of emotions evoked in the course of clinical work.

Emotional Expression Art Reflection

1. Begin a gratitude journal in which you weekly create an image, write a list, or write a poem about that for which you are uniquely grateful during the week.
2. Write a gratitude letter to a person who believed in you, encouraged you, or mentored you. This should be someone whom you have not adequately thanked and whom you can visit to read the letter. When the letter is complete, make a date to see the person and share your appreciation.
3. In response to an emotional situation regarding a client, create an image, song, poem or another type of writing. The art or writing can help you reflect on what you are feeling and what appropriate response might

be necessary for your well-being. Create a second, response image, to express the reparative urges. Share your art with a trusted friend, colleague, supervisor, or therapist who can help you deepen your understanding of it and its message for your life.

Questions for Self-Reflection

1. Do you take time to broaden and build the positive emotions that occur in your life? How could you better share gratitude or celebrate what went well in a day?
2. Do you have a regular time for sharing your feelings and thoughts about your professional work with a trusted supervisor, mentor, or peer?
3. What regular practice do you already use to engage in self-reflection? How is it working? Is there any way that this practice can be enhanced to better support you?

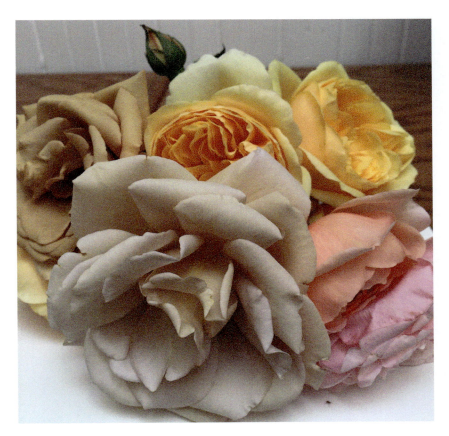

Plate 1 Sharing the Beauty of Sensation

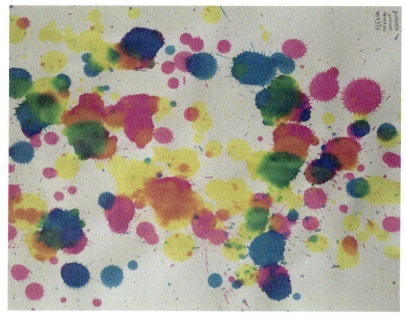
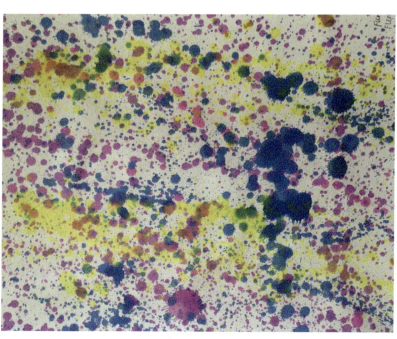

Plates 2 and 3 Art as a Vehicle for Movement and Stress Release

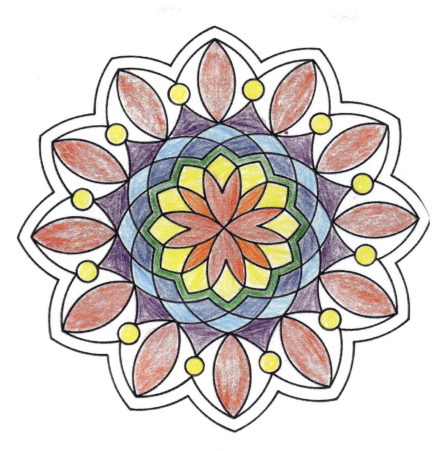

Plate 4 Mandala Coloring for Stress Reduction

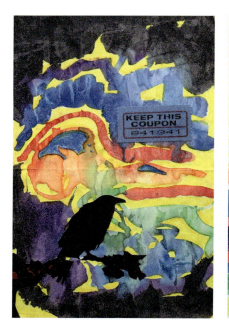 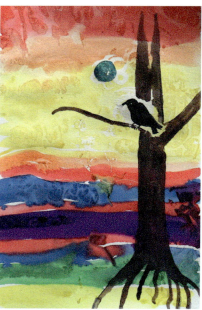

Plates 5 and 6 Emotion Expressed through Imagery

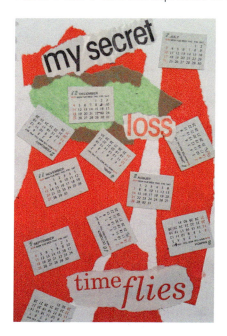 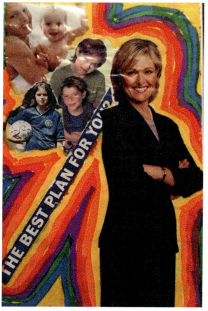

Plates 7 and 8 Collage: Evaluating Work-Life Balance

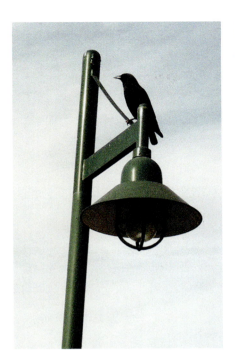

Plate 9 Animal Encounter: The Crow That Would Not Be Ignored

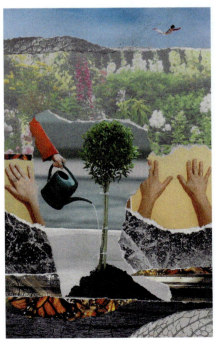

Plate 10 Collage: What it Takes to Nurture Creativity

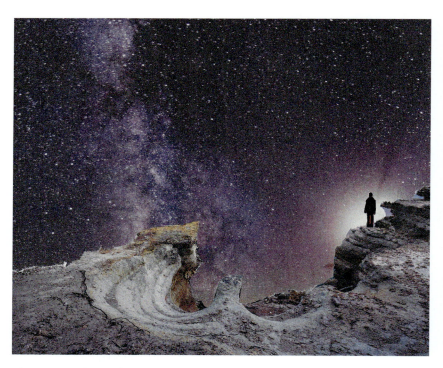

Plate 11 Collage of Awe and Wonder

Life Enrichment through Intellect

8

*The only means of strengthening one's intellect is to make up one's mind about nothing,
to let the mind be a thoroughfare for all thoughts.*

John Keats (1899, p. 405)

Although most everything that we do results from a coordinated operation of the entire brain, research shows that some complex mental processes can be broken down into discrete functions in specialized areas (Caeyenberghs & Leemans, 2014). Therefore, the Life Enrichment Model breaks down sophisticated cerebral processes into predominately left- and right-hemisphere brain functioning. The intellect component of the LEM is associated with left-hemisphere executive functioning that includes planning, problem solving, decision-making, cause-and-effect thinking, and delay of gratification. These brain functions tend to be slow and effortful, and are contrasted with the fast and intuitive processes on the other side of this component and the right hemisphere of the brain. The LEM provides a visual reminder that the intellect component is only one of several through which we take in, process, and express information. This chapter concerns enhancing left-brain activities to create dynamic balance with the right-brain processes discussed in Chapter 9.

Left-brain cognitive processes are emphasized in our educational system because they tend to be language-oriented, linear, and logical. This manner of thinking is indispensible for living an enriched life. Engaging in linear thought means that people can think through a sequence of events and determine the possible consequences of their actions, allowing them to rationally plan and prepare a course of action in order to ensure that events they can control run smoothly. When using left-brain processes, people are cool-headed and able to prepare a proactive response to challenges. This chapter will explore how logical deliberation allows people to change and replace cognitions that are no longer adaptive, and to increase affirmations of new life-enriching traits and behaviors. It will explain how changing the quality of self-talk and the internal narrative can be life enhancing, and how thoughtfully employed left-brain processes can help people achieve a sense of meaning in their work and increase professional satisfaction. Finally, this chapter will describe the ways in which leisure activities can enrich our lives through various intellectual pursuits.

Changing Thoughts

Increasing Positive Aspects of the Self-Narrative

Everyone develops a self-narrative or internal life story that explains the events of their lives. According to Ginot (2012), self-narratives are not merely beliefs about the self, but "an entire schema or self-state with its unique emotional tones, physical sensations, cognitions, as well as implicit and explicit attachment memories" (p. 60). As such, self-narratives are replete with substance and detail; they can be difficult to alter. However, to live an enriched life, it is necessary to examine any self-limiting aspects of the current life story and make adjustments that will lead to thriving rather than merely surviving. Using images can help people move away from "label-locked thinking" or the language-oriented labels that reduce people to the set of symptoms that diagnoses like "depression" or "autism" convey. Using images increases descriptive thinking and can reduce or remove self-stigma and handicapping self-descriptions (Grandin & Panek, 2013). Art can be used to examine and change outdated beliefs that no longer serve us (Steele & Kuban, 2012). This can be done to reframe childhood events, to examine the effects of vicarious trauma or professional burnout, and to strengthen investment in personal values and strengths – all of which can increase life enrichment.

One method of exploring, expanding, and transforming the life story is through creating a pictorial lifeline. This can be done as a cartoon or graphic novel in which important life events are depicted in panels and compiled into a single storyboard or entire book (Barry, 2014). A "lifeline" also can be created as an actual pen stroke that begins on the left side of a paper with birth and travels to the right side of the paper though the ups and downs of one's entire life. Significant highs and lows can be noted in words or images, and a narrative can be written to accompany the graph. As the last chapter revealed, an innate negativity bias means that most people tend to give more weight to negative events than positive ones, so it is possible that painful or stressful events could unduly influence one's life story. The graphic lifeline can allow the creator to achieve psychological distance from negative events and put them into a new perspective. This distance permits the creator to view harmful experiences more abstractly and less personally, creating space for an intentional shift in the self-narrative. Reflecting on the graphic lifeline can ultimately allow people to put greater weight on neutral and positive life events, while recognizing the personal strengths they cultivated through some of the negative events.

Increasing Self-Affirmation

Self-affirmation has been described as an integral part of the "psychological immune system," which occurs when an individual calls upon internal resources to reinforce their own sense of self and cope with challenges (Gilbert, Pinel, Wilson, Blumberg, & Wheatley, 1998). Self-affirmation is a process whereby people reflect on their core values and signature strengths (Harris, 2011) and in doing so enhance positive qualities like determination, self-control, and healthy habits. Self-affirmation can provide people with the ability to take a wider view of their lives and more effectively think through the effects of their current activities on long-term interests (Harris, 2011). When people are more invested in their long-range outcomes, they are more likely to discriminate between healthy and unhealthy behaviors, and to choose healthy ones. According to Gilbert, et al. (1998), a simple way to engage in self-affirmation is to rank order a list of one's core values and then write an essay about the top value, including why this is the most important value and a time when the value played a significant role in guiding behavior. Taking the time to reflect on core values and signature strengths offers people the opportunity to appreciate their unique personality traits and potentially reframe adverse life experiences, increasing engagement and life enrichment overall (Seligman, 2011).

Joan (pseudonym), a former client of mine, was the adult child of an alcoholic mother for whom she had cared for most of her life. From the age of 11 years old when her father left the home, Joan made meals and cleaned the house. She put her mother to bed most nights and comforted her when she cried about being alone. At the age of 27, Joan came to therapy because she was feeling sad and trapped by the circumstances of her life. Joan was not yet enrolled in graduate school as she had planned, but was stuck in a receptionist job, feeling that she could not let her boss down by cutting her hours to attend graduate school or by moving on to a new part-time job. Through engaging in the self-affirmation activity above, Joan was able to appreciate the determination, persistence, and self-control she had developed early in life, which would be essential for helping her apply to and complete graduate school. Realizing her strengths was the first step towards completing the applications, communicating changing career goals with her boss, and moving on with her life.

Developing Self-Compassion

In 2003, psychologist Kristin Neff introduced the Buddhist concept of self-compassion to Western psychology and, since then, it has since gained a great deal of professional and popular attention. Self-compassion is different from self-esteem, which relies on others' evaluations of the self, and from self-respect and self-efficacy, which are predominately related to self-evaluation or self-judgment. According to Neff (2003, p. 87), self-compassion:

> involves being touched by and open to one's own suffering, not avoiding or disconnecting from it, generating the desire to alleviate one's suffering and to heal oneself with kindness. Self-compassion also involves offering nonjudgmental understanding to one's pain, inadequacies and failures, so that one's experience is seen as part of the larger human experience.

Self-compassion is a way of viewing and interacting with the self that adopts a much kinder perspective and manner of self-talk than is common. Many people have a negative internal voice that is harshly critical and condemning of mistakes. Due to the ongoing stream of negative self-talk characteristic of this unforgiving "inner critic," new experiences can be inhibited and psychological growth stifled (Stone & Stone, 1993). Developing a self-compassionate internal voice is an effective way to counter the inner critic; to change the voice into one that is kind and concerned, eliciting soothing self-talk. From a place of kindness, life is rich with new possibilities (Hanson & Hanson, 2018).

The three elements of self-compassion are: (1) talking to yourself in the same kind and concerned way that you would talk to a friend; (2) realizing that everyone makes mistakes and not judging yourself harshly on the basis of perceived inadequacies; and (3) putting negative events into perspective, recognizing that one negative event is merely a single episode in an otherwise good life. Self-compassion has consistently been correlated with psychological and physical well-being – cultivating a compassionate inner voice has been shown to increase openness to new experiences, build safe and supportive social connections, and widen one's worldview to include a confident self (Barnard & Curry, 2011). Self-confidence, supportive relationships, and a curious mind are critical aspects of an enriched life.

Enhancing Meaning

Living with a sense of meaning is essential for life enrichment (Seligman, 2011). The typical meaning-making systems in which people engage to make sense of their lives are made up of three elements: First, a meaningful life is defined by coherence or understanding. A meaningful life is one that makes sense to us; we know why it is important to us and these precepts guide us. Second, a meaningful life is characterized by aims and goals that keep people focused. Last, a sense of significance creates meaning in our lives. One must feel that the life they are living has importance to the self, the community, and the world more broadly (Martela & Steger, 2016; Park, Currier, Harris, & Slattery; 2017). Feeling that coherence, direction, and significance describe one's vocation provides a sense of purpose that can outweigh many potentially harmful aspects of difficult work and provide a sense of life enrichment. Meaning and purpose are two elements that help replenish the deep well of psychological resources and spirituality supporting the excellent therapist. Indeed, the ability to engage in meaning-making is related to post-traumatic growth rather than post-traumatic stress disorder (Seligman, 2011).

Even though working as a helping professional can lead to the development of secondary traumatic stress, compassion fatigue, and burnout, developing one of these debilitating conditions is not a predetermined outcome. The development and internalization of life meaning can support post-traumatic growth instead. Seligman (2011) suggests that people reflect on a situation in which they have grown from adversity and write about it. In considering post-traumatic growth, it is beneficial to focus on three aspects: (1) how interpersonal relationships have improved; (2) how one's view of the self has been enhanced; and (3) how one's life philosophy has changed. Active consideration through left-hemisphere, effortful thought is encouraged because it increases the likelihood that adverse experiences will be accommodated into a new worldview and that psychological growth will result. The alternative is to assimilate the deleterious experiences into an existing worldview without deliberate thought, thus limiting the possibility for growth (Forgeard, et al., 2014).

People report that after deliberately thinking through challenging life experiences, they develop a greater appreciation for their relationships with friends and family, and desire greater intimacy in those relationships. They say that they perceive themselves in a more positive light: as wiser, more capable and more resilient in the face of stress. Finally, people who have grown from trauma often say that they have a more mindful and grateful approach to life, uniquely appreciating what each experience has to offer (Joseph, Murphy, & Regel, 2012; Tedeschi & Calhoun, 1996).

People who achieve a deep sense of meaning about their professional lives believe that their work goes beyond "doing a job" or "having a career" and extends to having a calling (Kelley & Kelley, 2013; Smith, 2016). Their daily work constantly challenges their professional knowledge and pushes them towards improvement; at the same time, they are able to master the work for optimal results (Csikszentmihalyi, 2008). People with a stimulating work life feel that that their unique strengths and abilities are utilized and appreciated. Their work meaningfully enriches their lives: there are definite goals to achieve and problem-solving strategies to try, evaluate, alter, and re-implement. Although challenged, they feel capable, masterful, and enlivened by a job well done (Csikszentmihalyi, 2008). Ongoing professional development, including relevant job training, and high-quality continuing education courses can augment this sense of vocational achievement (Harrison & Westwood, 2009). People who live an enriched life ensure that their knowledge and skills are growing in the context of their meaningful work. In doing so, they rate themselves not only as more satisfied with their work but also as more satisfied in their personal lives as well (Molino, Ghislieri, & Cortese, 2013).

Maintaining satisfaction with work also requires that people achieve a satisfying work–life balance. In most cultures, work–life balance is positively correlated with both life satisfaction and job satisfaction (Haar, Russo, Suñe, & Ollier-Malaterre, 2014). It is important for therapists to remember that there might be aspects of work over which they have no control, and to focus on the aspects that they can change, along with how their lives are enriched by activities and events outside of work. In addition, therapists should keep in mind that work–life balance changes over time with varying life demands. To maintain a satisfying work–life balance requires regular evaluation of shifting personal and professional demands. Using art is one way to examine the various roles and levels of satisfactions. Plates 7 and 8 are two images created by a woman who, in Plate 7, demonstrated her sense that her work life was getting out of hand; time was flying, not allowing her to enjoy her children. Plate 8 shows how she resolved to create better work–life boundaries so that she could increase enjoyable time with her children. The latter image was the first step towards implementing better boundaries and experiencing better balance.

Curiosity and Learning at Work

Learning something new is a cognitively enriching activity, which can occur in the form of continuing education to enrich professional skills and increase meaning derived from one's career. This may be an opportunity to seek out mentorship from someone who is also ready for innovation and inspiration and therefore is willing to take on additional training or supervision.

By taking on new skills or duties at work, you may be able to gently nudge your job in a different direction and change the course of your career. In my first job as a clinical psychologist at the University of Louisville Student Counseling Center, I took on the responsibility of supervising a student from the art therapy program. No one in the counseling center had supervised an art therapy student before, but I was interested in the opportunity to learn a new skill and appreciated that the art therapy faculty provided regular supervision to those who were not art therapists. The experiences of supervising in art therapy proved life-changing for me. I was enamored of the field and returned to graduate school to pursue additional training. Three years later I became a registered art therapist, and I continue to be enriched by my work every day.

Someone recently asked me what one of my favorite transformative moments was in working with art therapy clients. One moment did not stand out from the rest. What stood out was that this profession continues to enchant and enrich me as much today as it did when I was first learning about it. It affords me the opportunity to learn, grow, and travel as I teach in both new and familiar locations which never would have been possible if I had not taken a chance on those additional responsibilities.

Leisure Pastimes

Learning does not have to be limited to professional education; it can occur in a multitude of domains that lead equally to life enrichment. In my work at the Lifestyle Medicine Institute, I ask people about their hobbies and commonly encounter those whose only leisure activity is watching television. Many are genuinely puzzled as to why they should develop interests outside of work and even more so about how to go about doing it. The "why" question is answered easily: hobbies increase opportunities for learning. A curious and active mind is a significant aspect of an enriched life. Studies show that in the active learning phase, neuroplasticity occurs, which changes the structure of neurons, increases the number of synapses between neurons, and grows new neuronal connections. All of these structural changes in the brain allow neurons to send and receive information faster; thus, you will feel and be cognitively sharper. Learning to speak a foreign language or play a musical instrument are both associated with tremendous life-enriching cognitive benefits, including offsetting the onset of Alzheimer's disease (Bak, Nissan, Allerhand, & Deary, 2014; Levitin, 2007). Research has demonstrated that people who engage in continuous, active learning throughout their lives show greater abilities to cope with stress, increased self-esteem, and a greater sense of hope and purpose. Initiating goals for self-directed learning engenders feelings of achievement when milestones are met (Seligman, 2011). Thus, learning new skills and developing new hobbies has physical, mental and emotional benefits that are significantly life enriching.

The "how" question – how do I develop a hobby – is harder to answer, but I often tell people to consider engaging in a hobby that they enjoyed when they were young. What did they love to do when they were in sixth grade, before high school when they made their choice of vocational or college prep courses? Making these academic choices often focuses not only the course of study, but also the subsequent course of outside interests. Did you have a pastime that you let lapse because you got busy with homework and then with life? What you used to love to do might be fundamentally related to who you are. Did you like to ride a bike, play an instrument, crochet, or kayak? Try doing one of those things again as one way to enrich your life with a hobby.

Fostering Grit

Grit is a quality defined by a combination of passion and perseverance that characterizes successful people (Duckworth, 2016). Research demonstrates that more than academic or emotional intelligence, successful people demonstrate the ability to be persistent in setting and reaching goals. A sense of accomplishment is significantly related to well-being (Seligman, 2011), perhaps because achievement builds self-esteem. A solid sense of self-esteem is another essential component of an enriched life. According to Duckworth, developing grit relates to having a "growth mindset" or believing that change is possible. A person with a growth mindset learns from mistakes, knowing that failure is not a fixed condition. Duckworth recommends that to build grit, people practice doing one "hard thing" on a regular basis. This undertaking will be something that is difficult, which provokes failure but through continued efforts is improved upon. Setting aside time for self-reflection is necessary in order to grow grit and self-confidence, allowing for space to analyze setbacks and internalize successes.

Sharing Learning

Learning a new skill or content area often takes place in a class or formal course; to find classes you can look at the course listings at a local community college, professional network, or community center. But formal classes are not necessary for learning. Friends or colleagues can set up informal study groups where they equally contribute to the research, lecture, and discussion involved in learning. Book clubs meet to share and discuss what they have learned from their reading. It is common for book clubs to meet and discuss a book that everyone has read; in alternate book clubs, each member discusses their reading of a different book on a shared topic. Discussing ideas and challenging others stimulates creativity and increases well-being. Learning with other people strengthens relationships built on common interests, and can be a good way to increase motivation to engage in a new activity.

Summary and Conclusions

This chapter highlighted left-hemisphere cognitive processes which, in dynamic balance with the right-hemisphere processes described in the next chapter, are the most complex types of life-enriching experiences. Focusing on the intellect component of the Life Enhancement Model can help you develop various types of executive functioning skills. Left-hemisphere processes can permit you to re-evaluate your self-narrative and highlight the positive aspects of it. Changing the typical self-narrative and engaging in self-affirmation can reduce the innate negativity bias and decrease self-limiting beliefs. Cultivating a self-compassionate inner voice can increase self-acceptance and self-confidence. It is important to remember that coming from a place of kindness and concern towards the self is not self-pity or self-indulgent; it permits people to invest in, rather than shy away from, unfamiliar experiences. Reduced self-imposed negativity will support a new level of openness to life-enriching ideas and experiences. Diverse learning experiences can occur through work or leisure and can be that "one hard thing" that increases grit to further promote personal growth.

Working with the intellect component can help you identify positive character strengths, and their progression can be encouraged through the use of art and expressive writing. Reflection on the rewards and challenges of your professional life can foster meaning and add a sense of purpose that can outweigh the potentially harmful effects of working as a helping professional. Deliberate, thoughtful examination, and the affirmation of one's role and responsibilities as a therapist can help promote the development of internal resources which you can call upon to cope with challenges.

Intellect and Art Reflection

1. Draw a lifeline that begins on the left side of a long paper with your birth and travels to the right side of the paper through the ups and downs of your life. Mark significant highs and lows in words or images and write a narrative about the life you depicted to accompany the graph. Ask yourself whether more weight is given to negative events than positive ones and how it might be possible to change this interpretation of your life story. Could increasing a self-compassionate voice be a part of the change?
2. Create a collage that demonstrates the pros and cons of doing the professional work that you have chosen. If the cons outweigh the pros, is it time to look for a different position? If so, what steps can you take to move in a more positive direction? You might try creating a second image that develops the pro side of the collage into the next position or creating a skills-based résumé to think outside of the present job description.
3. Create an image that expresses one of your favorite things to do as a child. As you reflect upon the created image, think of a way to get back in touch with the activity that you used to love.

Questions for Self-Reflection

1. Engage in self-affirmation by rank-ordering a list of your core values and then writing an essay about the top value, including why this is your most important value and a time when this value played a significant role in guiding your behavior.
2. To increase your sense of accomplishment write about a proud achievement and detail the skills and abilities that you demonstrated by going about it.
3. To highlight meaning, either professionally or personally, write about a time when you grew from adversity. Make sure to include how your view of the world, yourself, and your important relationships were enriched by the experience.

Life Enrichment through Symbolism

9

*An idea, in the highest sense of that word,
cannot be conveyed but by a symbol.*
Samuel Taylor Coleridge (1853, p. 266)

In the Life Enrichment Model, "symbolic thinking" refers to what we typically think of as right-hemisphere cerebral processes. Chapter 8 described that left-hemisphere processes are language oriented and logical; they deal with factual information that tends to be fixed and singular in meaning. Right-hemisphere processes deal with information that is fluid and can contain multiple meanings. In addition, these processes have been described as holistic because they allow people to grasp the entire meaning of something, and even multiple layers of meaning, at once. They can help people organize large amounts of information simply and efficiently through the use of symbols. Right-brain thinking allows for the apprehension of meaning in a holistic and intuitive way rather than in a sequential and logical way. Intellect and symbolism work in dynamic balance to provide information, knowledge, and wisdom.

Symbolic thinking is emotional and spiritual; it typically emphasizes images and visual ways of thinking. This type of cognitive process occurs without deliberate effort; rather it is instinctive and occurs in flashes of insight or what Kahneman (2011) referred to as "fast thinking." However, when people look into what makes up fast or intuitive thought, it is clearly based on the accumulation of personal experience. The more experience one has with a subject, the more likely it is that whole meanings can be grasped in an instant and connection between topics, events, or people can be noticed and appreciated. When we are open to possibility, multiplicity of meaning, and fluidity of thought, all provide for tremendous life enrichment.

Symbolic thought can be personally meaningful – an image, poem, or ritual can have distinct meaning for an individual – or it can be universal, such that others can understand and relate to the meaning without providing detailed explanations. A universal symbol takes on meaning through shared history, culture, race, or social group, and can unite people in a common cause. The crucifix is a universal symbol of Christ's suffering which conveys multiple meanings to Christian people throughout the world. A personal symbol gains its significance through specific context: a momentous event in a person's life, a meaningful interaction with another person, a milestone reached. Recognizing and celebrating the significance of symbols is a way to enrich life by deepening connection and meaning.

Symbolic thinking is fluid and flexible, not fixed on a particular meaning as a left-brain label would be. Flexible thinking can be metaphorical, which allows meaning to develop on multiple levels. When Aristotle wrote "One swallow does not a summer make," he was not only referring to an actual bird not being a harbinger of a season, but also observing that one instance of any event does not necessarily portend the phenomenon. He used subtle language to warn people not to jump to conclusions. Thus, metaphor can enrich people's lives by allowing for the discussion of controversial or troubling subjects on many levels at once. It often is easier to approach difficult topics using figurative language. For example, I treated a patient with a substance use disorder who could talk much more easily about the "black bear" – her metaphor for addiction – than she could about her actual condition. Using the metaphor provided her freedom to examine the powerful grip of addiction: the fear and anguish she experienced were evident in the wild bear metaphor in ways for which she otherwise could not find words.

Using metaphor allows people to address difficult topics in language that is inclusive, descriptive, and emotional without being inflammatory. Symbolic thought is multidimensional and can include numerous connotations and emotions at the same time. It is multileveled; depending on the context, one meaning might be primary at one time, and other times, a different meaning takes precedence. Using symbolism allows people to project themselves into possibility and retrieve new significance. Through immersing themselves in the universal story, individuals can be enlivened and emerge with new, unique, and personally meaningful associations. Diverse associations are particularly evident and accessible in the visual arts because the multiple interpretations are more obvious in images than they are in language and other forms of expression.

Art

Participation in the arts allows people to experience various delightful, daring, or dangerous aspects of life from a safe distance. These experiences are life enriching without risk, and provide numerous benefits. Visiting museums has been shown to increase critical thinking skills (Bowen, Greene, & Kisida, 2014), perhaps because all of the relationships among elements in artworks are not spelled out logically but are intuited. Furthermore, as each new image is encountered, an active and intuitive process is generated that builds on previous experience with personal and universal symbols. As Ernst Fischer wrote in his 1959 book, *The Necessity of Art*, "Art in its origins was magic, a magic aid towards mastering a real but unexplored world" (p. 13). I would add that art is an aid in mastering two worlds. It allows us to explore and understand both the outer world as well as our own inner world. Additionally, engaging in symbolism allows for the simultaneous encountering of known and unknown aspects of the self and the world.

Helping Professionals take note: Visit a museum or art gallery and immerse yourself in the work of a particular artist, artistic movement, or a period in art history that interests you. Allow all of the associations that occur to enrich your view of yourself, your world, and your future.

We can also use art to examine and change the old, outdated beliefs by which we live our lives (Steele & Kuban, 2012). In his classic work, *The Necessity of Art*, Ernst Fischer explained that when primitive people created tools, "a new power over nature had been gained, and this power was potentially unlimited. In this discovery lay one of the roots of magic, and therefore, of art" (1959, p. 19). Indeed, art has been used through the ages for purposes of magical self-exploration, illumination, and expansion. From ancient times, through the Renaissance, to the present time, art has illuminated Western religion. In the 12th century, religious mystic and teacher Hildegard of Bingen used art to illuminate spiritual visions and explain a complex religious philosophy (Fox, 2002). The experience of viewing or creating visual art allows people to experience the mysterious and the divine, even in the absence of logical understanding. Art is a means through which to experience the self in relation to the universe. It provides a means to express the imagination in ways that are not tied to the rather fixed formality of language and therefore increases the possibility of personal self-expression (Fischer, 1959).

Viewing and creating art are life-enriching activities that can be available to individuals at all times. Although people tend to save up their art viewing time for museum visits, the ability to view art in books, online, and in our homes means that these compelling experiences are always available. People decorate their homes with art to stimulate and enrich their lives, yet the inspiration lessens over time because people habituate to the same artworks displayed in the same places. When people no longer actively observe their art, it has less power to enrich. However, all that is required is to move a painting to another location or put a sculpture in an unfamiliar place: Suddenly it is new again, containing all of its original influence to enchant and enrich.

Helping Professionals take note: Switch up the art you have in your home to ensure it remains actively inspirational. See your art with new eyes and it will greatly enrich your life.

When people view personally meaningful art, it activates parts of the brain that include reward centers as well as self-referential or autobiographical thought (Chatterjee, 2015; Vessel, Starr, & Rubin, 2002). Neuroscientists have taken this to mean that viewing art is not a passive activity but an active one, which derives from the integration of sensory and emotional responses resulting in unique personal meaning. The activity of viewing art leads to self-referential thought that can provoke learning about the self and the relationship of the self to the larger world. Of course, creating art also triggers the same processes and can be life enriching in a symbolic way. In addition, art allows people to express all parts of themselves, and this well-rounded view can encourage acceptance of previously disliked or disowned parts of the self (Hinz, 2009).

This book is full of suggestions for enhancing personal meaning through the use of art. And if you want to create, you do not have to wait until you have an hour or two blocked off. Making art can happen in an instant; it can be as simple as editing photos on your smartphone, tablet, or computer. It can include creating Artist Trading Card-sized doodles, or using stamps or washi tape to enhance a previously created postcard. In fact, making art for others is a creative way to say that you care – a way to engage in self-care and care for others at the same time.

Sharing Symbols: Rituals

Embodying metaphor in action can result in ritual. A ritual is a physical act or ceremony, usually commemorating a momentous occasion, done in a prescribed way or according to social custom (Rossner & Meher, 2014). In the Western world, we live in a relatively ritually deprived society; we do not have a great deal of ceremony outside of some national holidays and even then, attendance at rites or rituals is not mandatory so many people do not participate. For example, in the United States, Memorial Day is a federal holiday in which our nation honors those who have lost their lives serving their country in the armed forces. Many people take a trip over the long Memorial Day weekend that does not involve honoring servicemen and women. Although there are not a great number of shared national rituals in the United States, we do have lesser rituals that can add enrichment to our lives if we engage in them mindfully.

A ritual practice can aid the transition from work to home as a new phase of the day is initiated. Researchers have divided the "micro transition" between work and home into exiting work, transition space, and entering home. Much of the time these transitions go unnoticed and carryover effects from work to home are common. Rituals inserted at any point can aid temporal, physical, psychological, or social transitions and clarify the boundaries between work and home (Ashforth, Kreiner, & Fugate, 2000). A ritual at end of the work day signals a job well done. Some people set aside 15–30 minutes at the end of the day to recap what went well and begin a plan for the next day. Creating lists can be a significant part of the ritual; the lists, and therefore work concerns, are left at the office. Commuting time can be a buffer between roles and aid in work–home transition. Time on public transportation can be mindfully engaging as time to contemplate and time to decompress, thus aiding psychological transition. Walking or riding a bike can aid transition with a physical release of tension. Rituals at home signal engagement with loved ones. The entry door can be a signal or carry a message about the meaning of family. In addition, the ritual of greeting each family member and pet immediately upon entering the house continues the social transition. Other ways to aid the transition are changing clothes, taking a walk, and lighting a candle. Sharing rituals with others can heighten their meaning and ability to enrich people's lives.

Social and Religious Rituals

Everyday social rituals include sharing music, dance, sports, coffee, wine, kisses, and handshakes. When we participate mindlessly, these rituals frequently go unnoticed. For example, if I meet someone without really engaging, I will forget the person's name within minutes. Yet, if I interact mindfully, grasping my new friend's hand firmly, looking her in the eye and repeating her name; if I remember that our right hands are clasped so that our hearts, on the left side of our chests, are open to one another; I will remember the name of this person, my new friend. Religious rituals express reverence for a deity or idealized state of humanity, but there is no guarantee that I participate mindfully in the associated rites or sacraments. If I enter into my church absent-mindedly and hurriedly take communion, it does not make an impact on my life. On the other hand, if I am focused when I enter my church and thoughtfully and reverently receive communion, this ritual will enrich my life.

Family Rituals

Family rituals have the power to bond family members together with common memories, values, and pleasure. In my household, we have a simple ritual at our disposal every evening in the form of the family dinner. Families who eat dinner together report greater overall satisfaction with their lives. As I wrote in Chapter 4, sharing the family meal has been shown to protect against the development of negative behaviors in children and adolescents (Fishel, 2015). The family meal is a time to talk about the day, share anecdotes and feelings, and solve problems. It also can be an opportunity for an enriching ritual encounter. For example, some families have a "special plate" ritual added to the family meal where family members are recognized and celebrated for their accomplishments. On any given day a distinctive plate at the table (in some families it is a red plate) denotes that the chosen family member has something out of the ordinary to share. That person receives extra "air time" to discuss the special event or achievement.

The family meal can just be fun as children and adults share memories and stories. Sharing in this way creates the family lore that bonds relatives together. Rituals in the form of family traditions also help enrich and build strong family bonds. If you have children, you know that all it takes to start a family tradition is do something the same way two or three times before you begin to hear, "we always do it this way." After a few weeks, Friday pizza and movie night can easily become a family tradition. Other family rituals include regular reunions for extended relatives, game nights (card games, board games, or outdoor games), and holiday activities including songs, artwork, trips, and foods.

More Experiences with Symbolism

Symbolism enriches people's lives by taking them out of the ordinary world and inviting them into one that includes the mysterious. It helps people go beyond what is logical and factual to explore ethereal concepts like beauty and love. Symbolism pulls individuals into that which they do not fully understand but that calls them to know more, be more, and experience more. Those places and experiences where people encounter universal symbols are fertile ground for evoking powerful enrichment. The remainder of this chapter will explore some of the avenues for experiencing universal symbols: reading myths and stories, appreciating illustrated books, reading or writing poetry, synchronicity, animal encounters and dreams.

Reading Myths and Stories

Each culture begins with a creation myth that tells the origin story and contains many other anecdotes relating to the history and character of its people. These tales define cultures and bind them together. Our own myths help us understand how and why certain things are important to us and why other things do not matter as much. Carl Jung would say that our myths allow us to be in touch with the "collective unconscious," helping us understand the symbols that call to us even when we do not consciously understand why we are drawn to them. This level of simultaneous knowing and not knowing is enriching if we embrace it and invite it to enrich our lives. For example, Joseph Campbell explains in *The Power of Myth* that Hero's Journey stories resonate with us because we have all had to overcome obstacles in our lives to achieve self-knowledge and self-acceptance (Campbell, 1991).

Myths and stories permeate the Bible and other sacred writing, helping us experience our religion and spirituality in a holistic and intuitive manner. Ancient people responded to myths and parables because they could immerse themselves in the stories and live the message of their religion through them. Today, writers like John O'Donohue in *To Bless the Space Between Us: A Book of Blessings* and David Whyte in *Consolations: The Solace, Nourishment and Underlying Meaning of Everyday Words* take us beyond ourselves into the realm of spirituality through the symbols available to us every day. Both books seem to me ideal companions for our busy lives because they contain short, isolated passages that can be read independently for inspiration, support, and enrichment.

Illustrated Books

One of my greatest pleasures when my children were young was accompanying them to the local public library and helping them select a pile of picture books to read together. I was just as engaged with the illustrated stories as they were, perhaps even more so because I could appreciate the technical skill and emotional investment of the artists. Unfortunately, publishers assume that adults' preferences change so that they are not interested in books with pictures; after middle school books usually do not contain illustrations. However, I continue to collect and appreciate adult storybooks, graphic novels, and other illustrated books for adults because the images inspire me. I particularly like *A Conference of the Birds* by Peter Sis. In this book the artist illustrated an ancient Persian myth and Hero's Journey. Graphic novels such as *Allison Bechdel's Are You My Mother?* relates a coming of age story through paneled stories, the pictures adding depth of emotion and propelling the story forward like a traditional comic book. Recently the field of "graphic medicine" has emerged to blend the endeavors of physicians, patients, and allied health professionals in telling the stories of different health and illness journeys through graphic means (King, 2017). Clearly, for this group of people, illustrations enrich their stories in ways that words alone do not. Graphic depictions deepen the story and enrich the experience.

Poetry

Reading or writing poetry is another symbolically enriching activity. Poets use symbolic language to convey personal and universal themes that can broaden or intensify experience. T.S. Eliot proclaimed that "genuine poetry can communicate before it is understood" (Eliot, 1964, p. 238). This means that people are able to intuit the significance of a poem before they understand it in a logical way. Thus, poetry speaks to individuals in a way that prose does not. Poems permit people to convey topics that are complicated or troublesome in language that is imaginative and lyrical. Like metaphor, poetry has the ability to carry multiple meanings, and thus appeals to different people for a variety of reasons. To add poetry to your life, you might pick up a volume at a used bookstore. If you thumb through the book and find a poem that you like, chances are there are more where that came from. Ask friends and mentors who their favorite poets are. The Poetry Foundation (www.poetryfoundation.org) offers a free smartphone app that functions as a random poem generator. The app can introduce you to modern and classic verses for inspiration and enrichment.

Synchronicity, Animal Encounters, and Dreams

Synchronicity is a concept that Carl Jung introduced to explain the confluence of seemingly random events that appear to have a meaningful and causal connection. Jung defined synchronicity as "meaningful coincidence" and proposed that these encounters offered significant connections to our deeper selves (Forrer, 2015). Appreciating coincidence connects us to a world of infinite possibilities. One type of synchronic event can occur when we encounter an animal in our life that makes us pause and consider it. Once I was having lunch with a friend who had lost her husband two years prior. After lunch, a crow was sitting on a lamp post in the parking lot cawing loudly; it would not be ignored. I took the picture of it shown in Plate 9, and when I got home, looked up the symbolism of the crow. I found that the crow is celebrated for its intelligence and resiliency; it is a symbol of flexibility and adaptability. I read that when it appears in someone's life, the crow can be a sign that change is coming or a new beginning is possible. When I thought about what the synchronistic animal encounter might mean to my friend and me, it seemed that the crow heralded a new era: Its insistent appearance was saying that it was okay for my friend to move on with her life without her husband; the change that was coming could be a welcome one.

Dreams also can also provide important messages if individuals pay attention. It is not necessary to be an expert in interpreting dreams to gain information from them, but it is necessary to be open to the world of infinite possibilities. People encounter so many experiences and so much information during the day that they cannot process all of it consciously. Therefore, the brain scrambles the details, people, and places and serves them up at night in dream form. If people pay attention to a dream sequence or even just a dream fragment, they can gain new and significant information. Dreams are where universal figures are met, so it can help to know something about these characters and what their prescribed message might be. Looking up an article or book about archetypal symbols is a good starting place.

Summary and Conclusions

Symbolic, right-brain thinking is holistic, intuitive, visual, and spiritual. It allows people to apprehend significance in flashes of insight and to convey meaning through metaphor. Life is enhanced through embracing mystery, contemplating multiple layers of meaning, and engaging in critical thinking, all of which are improved through participation in the arts. Using art as a method of personal or universal self-expression can facilitate these right-hemisphere processes in our brain and further enrich our experiences. Life is richer when we are able to consider multiple layers of meaning around a single concept. Metaphor can be embodied in ritual and people's lives made richer through mindful participation in social, family, and religious encounters. Deliberate and mindful participation in rituals that help with the transition between work and home can promote detachment from work and authentic re-engagement in home life. Tending to these transitions widens the margins between home and work and affords greater space and time for life enrichment.

This chapter introduced and discussed a range of enriching symbolic activities, including reading myths and stories and finding personal application for universal healing themes. Each represents a unique way to gain information that is intuitive and relevant and that connects us to unlimited life-enriching possibilities. Living with uncertainty and immersing ourselves in other people's stories are risk-free ways to encounter diverse points of view, values, and emotions. Encountering these universal themes in the forms of myths, art, poetry, and novels can allow us to acknowledge and embrace previously unknown or split-off parts of ourselves which can broaden and deepen our work as Helping Professionals.

Symbolism and Art Reflection

1. Pay attention to your dreams tonight and immediately upon waking, create an image of an entire dream sequence or just one part of a dream. As you contemplate the image, what does it tell you about yourself or your current life circumstances?
2. Create a self-portrait as a character from your favorite fairy tale. How is this character representative of a part of you?
3. Find three images from a magazine that appeal to you and combine them in a small collage. Remaining open to the world of infinite possibilities, write about how these images represents a part of you.

Questions for Self-Reflection

1. What sorts of rituals do you engage in on a regular basis? Can you think of mindful ways to increase your participation in one of them and thus enrich your life?
2. Read the poem "The Journey" by Mary Oliver or "Love after Love" by Derek Walcott (full texts of both are available online) and reflect on how the message of the poem can enrich your life.
3. Is there an animal that has appeared in your life recently? Look up the symbolism of the animal and decipher how it might apply to you at this time in your life.

Life Enrichment through Creativity

10

> *Talent hits a target no one else can hit;*
> *Genius hits a target no one else can see.*
> Arthur Schopenhauer (1958, p. 391)

Many years ago, the terms "genius" and "creativity" often were used interchangeably, thus leading to the belief that creativity was an inborn talent reserved only for a small, elite group of people. However, the definition of creativity commonly used today in psychological research involves only two elements: originality and effectiveness (Runco & Jaeger, 2012). Accordingly, creativity has been described as the combination of things or ideas in ways that are perceived as both novel and useful. I like this definition of creativity because it is inclusive; it refutes the belief that creativity is a special skill available only to a privileged few. All people are creative, but they are creative in different ways and to different degrees. This inclusive definition of creativity can help all people celebrate their "everyday creativity" (Richards, 2014), or the ways in which they combine things or ideas in new and effective ways to enhance their lives.

The creative level of the Life Enrichment Model also emphasizes that when people are engaged in creative activities, the emphasis is on "putting it all together" or the integration of ideas, especially self-referential ideas and self-actualizing tendencies (Lusebrink, 1990). Based on his research, psychologist Mihaly Csikszentmihalyi popularized the idea that we can achieve self-actualization by finding a state of "flow" in our work or our hobbies (Csikszentmihalyi, 2008). Creative experiences allow us to enter the flow state.

Creativity and Flow

As described in Chapter 2, flow can be characterized as a very pleasurable state of focused attention that occurs when a person is challenged by an activity but, through concentrated effort, is able to master it (Csikszentmihalyi, 2008). When in flow, the concentrated effort is unforced, and the person feels one with the task, unlikely to become distracted or focus attention elsewhere. The type of activity that induces flow can vary from intensely physical to very intellectual; the common factors are that a person feels challenged, but masterful. When in flow, not only is a person uniquely attentive, but also is so absorbed in the task at hand that their normal perception of time is altered. Time seems to slow down remarkably or pass extraordinarily quickly.

Although they can sometimes be difficult to begin, we appreciate flow experiences because they are intrinsically engaging and rewarding. Being in flow is associated with feelings of great satisfaction and moments of peak joy (Csikszentmihalyi, 2008). These peak experiences are referred to as self-actualizing experiences. They occur when people feel that they are acting as their best possible selves. This manifestation of the best self elicits feelings of contentment during the task itself, and when people experience flow, the rest of their day is characterized by increased well-being. The long-lasting feelings of well-being that result from creative self-expression are a foundation for the enriched life.

Because engaging in flow activities increases overall and lasting well-being, exercising creativity can help prevent the negative conditions associated with the helping professions like secondary traumatic stress and compassion fatigue. It is important to remember how good it feels to engage in creative endeavors, and to note that engagement can be relaxing and invigorating at the same time. Further, creativity involves risk – putting things or ideas together in new ways can feel uncomfortable. Human beings are hard-wired to seek safety and often mistake comfort for safety, thus choosing the familiar over the unfamiliar or effortful. The majority of participants in the lifestyle medicine program where I work spend their evenings watching television, believing it is an entertaining and relaxing activity. However, when people closely examine the effects of television, they realize that it is not relaxing; it tends to be mindless and numbing when it is the default evening activity. This realization often prompts people to give up "binge watching" shows on video channels. Binge watching occurs easily because one show is cued up directly after another so that there is no break between them; audience members are hooked, unable to stop.

Then again, watching television can be more enriching than numbing; it can be entertaining and enlightening if people watch in a deliberate manner. Mindfully watching television can spark creative opportunities; it can increase knowledge or stimulate new ideas for cooking, decorating, travel, or sport. Mindful watching means that people choose programs that fit the occasion, watch deliberately chosen shows rather than channel surf, and limit the time in front of the television. One study showed that young adults who spent less time watching television showed better cognitive functioning as middle-aged adults than their peers who were heavy viewers (Hoang, et al., 2016).

Expert therapists report that to maintain their own well-being, they intentionally choose television programs or movies that enrich or distract them. They make a conscious decision not to engage with television shows that can re-enact the trauma that they experience during their work days (Mullenbach & Skovholt, 2001; Norcross & Guy, 2007). In addition, watching a carefully selected television program can be used as a well-deserved reward, encouraging mindful engagement with other tasks that must be completed first. I know people who do not watch television automatically, but only after they have achieved their fitness goals for the day. In summary, television watching, which is often our "default reward" at the end of a long day, can be made more relaxing and enriching with more attention to the viewing content and circumstances.

Creativity and Play

Television viewing is not highly rated when researchers ask people to track and rate their daily activities, levels of creativity, and moods. Increased creativity and positive mood are associated with being open to and having new experiences (Silvia, et al., 2014). Some researchers would call openness to new experiences and activity without agenda, "play." Psychologist Stuart Brown has spent his professional life studying the various types of play and their purposes (Brown, 2009). There are at least five different types of play (physical play, object play, rough and tumble play, spectator/ritual play, and imaginative play) which are first experienced during childhood and have varying effects on adult outcomes.

According to Brown, play is not just important for children; it is significant for adults because it encourages spontaneity, creativity, and positive mood. The relationship between positive mood, creativity and openness to new experience makes sense because openness to novel experience allows for the influx of innovative ideas and activities that are necessary elements of creativity. Also, everyday creativity has been shown to precede or activate other positive states including energy, enthusiasm, and engagement (Silvia, et al., 2014). Therefore, creativity can be considered a positive emotion regulation strategy (Kopcsó & Láng, 2017); engaging in creative activities can enhance your mood and increase passion and purpose.

According to the Life Enrichment Model, creative experiences can occur through experience with a single aspect of the model (e.g., movement only or intellect only) or they can involve the combination of various forms of experience. When a single element of the LEM is involved, the creative experience might be a spontaneous dance that is uniquely individual or some other singular experience. The expression does not have to be a masterpiece; it has to be personal and meaningful. However, creativity can also involve the combination of various forms of activity to provide a holistic experience for life enrichment that promotes and reinforces optimal health. For example, the person who knits a sweater is involved with soft and colorful yarn which is a sensuous experience, while the knitting itself is a motor experience as well. Finally, the knitter must follow a visual-spatial pattern to successfully complete the garment. At least three components of the LEM are involved in this creative endeavor.

Creativity and Psychological Growth

Whether one or more elements of the LEM are involved, creativity promotes either an experience of true expression of the known self, or the integration of new information that expands or deepens one's sense of self (Harter, 2007). Creative experiences help clarify thoughts and feelings about the self and promote psychological growth. According to Richards (2014), when people are engaged in creative activities they are keenly observant, non-defensive, collaborative, and brave. Creativity increases resiliency. In addition, creative activities increase agency and positive emotions; they bring about emotional balance and can increase behavioral options. Creative experiences can help people gain a positive perspective on an experience previously conceived as negative through the process of post traumatic growth (Forgeard, et al., 2014).

Creative experiences can help people think differently than they normally do, including thinking about themselves in a more positive way. Encouraging different views of the self can help build psychological capital, a positive state of psychological development that includes hope, optimism, self-efficacy, and resiliency (Dawkins, Martin, Scott, & Sanderson, 2013; Newman, Ucbasaran,

Zhu, & Hirst, 2014). Through either augmenting existing strengths, or improving perceived personal deficits, engaging in creative writing assignments can help people increase psychological capital (Meyers, van Woerkom, de Reuver, Bakk, & Oberski, 2015). Psychological capital is one of the elements that fills the deep well necessary to carry out excellent work as a helping professional. Feelings of hope, optimism, and self-efficacy promote compassion and will provide a firm foundation in resiliency.

Creativity and Connection

Research shows that working with other people enhances creativity (Kelley & Kelley, 2013; Lehrer, 2012). Creating with others adds ideas and broadens existing ones. Each solution that a person poses to a specific problem has the potential to encourage new ideas or solutions from other people in the group. Despite what conventional thought implies, many projects or activities benefit from having another critical set of eyes on them, even at the beginning or brainstorming stage. The popular belief about brainstorming is that all ideas are generated uncritically before they are discussed or judged, assuming that early judgment will shut down the generation of ideas and stifle creative thought. On the contrary, research has indicated that this sort of "critical collaboration" right at the beginning stimulates people to come up with even more creative options than uncritical brainstorming techniques (Lehrer, 2012). Engaging in creative activities with others builds solid bonds between people and produces better outcomes.

Not only does creativity bond people together, it also connects people to their highest self, their best possible self, or their creative self. Connection with the creative self can initiate profound self-acceptance and the building of psychological capital, as people feel better about themselves when they are reminded of their finest characteristics. Creativity can connect people to a higher power, or be used as a tool through which individuals can express their connection to a higher power. Contemplation of the fact that they were created by a divine or universal force can connect people with their own divine and creative capacities.

Increasing Creativity

Creativity is not a fixed condition of the mind – people can learn to cultivate creativity (Lehrer, 2012; Richards, 2014). In his 2012 *New York Times* bestselling book on creativity, *Imagine: How Creativity Works*, journalist Jonah Lehrer interviewed creative people from disparate fields and wrote fascinating accounts of their accomplishments. From his interviews, he culled suggestions about how to support greater creativity. Some of his suggestions include letting go, being an outsider, thinking like a child, collaboration, interacting with strangers and city living. "Letting go" refers to making time to relax and allow remote association to flow through the mind. It helps to have no pressing outside demands to attend to so that the mind can wander freely without interference from the "inner critic." If there is no specific task at hand, the inner critic can be quieted because there is nothing to criticize. In addition, letting your mind wander allows for the headspace needed to make the varied connections associated with creative, divergent thinking. As was mentioned in a previous chapter, contemplating a concept or object for a long period of time permits the secondary characteristics to surface, thus increasing the possibility of divergent thinking and creative potential (Arnheim, 1966).

Divergent thinking is associated with creativity because the more remote associations that are generated to an issue or problem, the more probable a novel and useful combination will emerge. This form of thinking is stimulated when a person is an "outsider" or existing in unfamiliar surroundings. Lehrer (2012) wrote that travel stimulates creativity because of the outsider effect. When people have to think about all manner of daily tasks that they usually take for granted (e.g., what subway route to take; what shop carries the needed items), many different thoughts and associations are stimulated that contribute to creativity. He wrote that people do not travel to Paris to write about Paris, they go to become stimulated to write. Even simple "outsider" experiences that happen in your own area can stimulate divergent thoughts and remote associations.

Helping Professionals take note: To spark the outsider effect in your own area, try going to a neighborhood that you do not normally frequent. If your city has ethnically diverse neighborhoods, go to a place where you will encounter foods, clothing, language, and sights that are not familiar. Notice the effects on your creative output.

Creativity also is enhanced when we interact with strangers, when we talk with people who come from different backgrounds and walks of life. People find opportunities to collaborate with strangers in community workshops and classes. Creativity will flourish when you volunteer to work with a person that you do not know at the next meeting you attend. Of course, chance encounters will happen if people travel, wander into neighborhoods that are not familiar, and talk with people at work who perform different job functions. Switching jobs with someone for a day or just taking on one of their tasks is another way to increase remote associations (Kelley & Kelley, 2013). It is likely that city living increases creativity because it involves both interactions with strangers and more frequent forays into unknown neighborhoods. When associations are loose and the mind is open to new possibilities, creativity is increased.

Creative experiences occur when people put things together in ways that are different and useful. People can increase their chances of experiencing everyday creative moments if they build, cook, or grow something that they have not before. Creative enrichment does not always require active production of art; it can include looking at or listening to various works of art. Looking at a painting by a master artist is a creative but arguably passive activity that can provoke self-reflection or self-affirmation (Vartanian & Skov, 2014). For example, at various times in their lives, people adopt special songs that are so personally meaningful that they increase motivation and provide inspiration. Listening to a favorite song represents the blending of many expressive elements to establish a complete and fundamentally enriching experience. A song involves rhythm and can make people move. Many songs are emotionally evocative because of their melodies, but additionally so because of their universally meaningful poetics. The combination of all three features can promote the song to a creatively enhancing theme song. Make sure to include music as an integral part of an enriched life.

In summary, all activities that increase opportunities for remote and loose associations can stimulate divergent thinking and heighten creativity. According to psychologist Rick Hanson, creativity and enrichment have an additive relationship with one another. Creativity helps enrich experience and enriched experience helps increase creativity. He suggested that to increase creativity, a person should first fully engage in an experience and enrich the experience by "making it bigger" or intensifying its unique aspects (exaggerating a movement, concentrating on a color). He then advised absorbing the experience by "receiving it" or making sure that the experience is savored to its fullest. Creativity and enrichment are further enhanced when people find reward in the experience. And finally, creativity is cultivated by linking the enriching experience to similar ones (Hanson, 2017).

It also boosts creativity to be surrounded by objects or images that stimulate diverse associations – things from various countries and of various uses. Looking at a diverse array of items will stimulate conscious and unconscious associations. The image displayed in Plate 10 is a collage about nurturing creativity. The woman who put together the collection of images was inspired by an array of images which caused many diverse associations.

She wrote of the image: What my creativity needs to blossom is solid fertile ground / light and air / water to nourish / hands that care. I need beauty around me/ butterfly wings / a blue sky to catch me / and tender saplings. Signs of transformation; silent revolution.

In addition to images or objects, various colors have been associated with increased creativity. The color blue has been shown to double divergent thoughts and problem solving, while red leads to more convergent thinking or converging on a single idea or solution (Mehta & Zhu, 2009). Green has been associated with increased creative thought, regardless of people's conscious associations to the color (Lichtenfeld, Elliot, Maier, & Pekrun, 2012).

Summary and Conclusions

The Life Enrichment Model holds to a definition of everyday creativity in which everyone is encouraged to honor the ways in which they combine things or ideas in ways that are original and effective to help enrich their lives. Creative experiences happen with building, cooking, and growing something that you have not before. Creativity is associated with the positive state of flow in which people are entirely absorbed in a task, lose track of time, and are greatly satisfied with the experience. Having creative flow experiences increases long-lasting feelings of well-being that are a foundation for the enriched life. Play is one way that people create space for creative activities, where they are open to new ideas and experiences. During play people act without an agenda which allows for the spontaneous production of ideas and events.

This chapter discussed the many positive effects of creative engagement, especially its ability to build psychological capital, the deep well that sustains excellent personal well-being and professional practice. Self-acceptance, belonging, and connection with a higher power all take place through the creative process. Connecting with the creative self enhances self-acceptance because people thrive on opportunities to be their best possible selves. This creative connection helps replenish the well of positive emotion, self-efficacy, and optimism that supports the excellent therapist. Creative experiences are especially enriching when they allow people to experience a moment of new insight about themselves or a moment of perfect self-expression. Group collaboration heightens creativity, as do situations where divergent thinking is encouraged such as letting go, being an outsider (even in your own town), interacting with strangers, travel, and working in groups. Make sure to prioritize creativity; invest your energy, time, and resources so that you can notice that you already do creative things every day.

Creativity and Art Reflection

1. Randomly chose one page from a magazine and tear it out. Imagine that this page contains and image or a word that is a special gift for you. Cut out the word or image and glue it to a new piece of paper. Add other elements to the image to develop this gift or write for ten minutes without regard for spelling, punctuation or grammar about how this is a unique and personal gift.
2. Create an image of the "inner muse" (Wilkinson & Chilton, 2017) which is the opposite of the inner critic. The inner muse is that internal part of you that loves and wants to create. Allow it to take form and then dialogue with it. Allow it to speak to you about how you are creative.
3. Create an image of what you need to nurture your creativity. Block out time on your calendar this week for a "play date" to express yourself creatively.

Questions for Self-Reflection

1. What times in your life have you acted spontaneously, without an agenda? Do you have unstructured time in your week where ideas can just occur?
2. What experiences in your day allow you to experience a state of flow: a challenging but engaging task in which you feel merged with the experience and lost in time? Pay attention to the long-lasting feelings of well-being that result from these flow experiences.

Living Optimally
A Deep Well, Wide Margins, and Firm Boundaries

11

> *There is only one good, the cause and the support of a happy life:*
> *to trust in ourselves.*
> Seneca the Younger (2016, p. 77)

As I introduced in Chapter 1, there are three essential pieces to living an enriched life, which also make up the foundation to sustaining an excellent therapy practice: a deep well, wide margins, and firm boundaries. When you live an enriched life, these concepts begin to play a bigger role in your daily routine because they build upon one another in virtuous cycles – enlivened by the practices the Life Enrichment Model suggests. The LEM provides a starting point for understanding and implementing the elements of an enriched life. As outlined in previous chapters, therapists can use the LEM to evaluate the sensual, physical, emotional, intellectual, symbolic, and creative aspects of their lives, and determine how they might be mindfully honored and enhanced to provide greater life enrichment.

The deep well consists of psychological resources, physical energy, and spiritual inspiration. This well provides the depth of empathic experience necessary in caring for others. To have wide margins means to have time built into the day for breaks. Sometimes a break is for distraction and sometimes it is for reflection, but when one is living mindfully, it is always necessary to have time between activities. Wide margins ensure time for mindful participation in self-reflection and creative practices, both foundations for excellent self-care and clinical practice. Finally, stable boundaries around personal and professional activities are central to an enriched life.

In order to embrace firm boundaries, therapists must realize that it is not selfish to focus on their own needs; it is self-preservation. When people live an enriched life, they enhance their physical health and have more energy to give to others. Good boundaries safeguard time for personal life enrichment practices that further refresh the deep well.

A Deep Well

Psychological capital is one of the elements that fills the deep well necessary to carry out excellent work as a Helping Professional. As was introduced in the last chapter, psychological capital is made up of hope, optimism, and self-efficacy. These feelings can promote compassion, especially directed towards the self, and provide a firm foundation in resiliency. Psychological capital has also been related to "positive growth initiative," which is a "positive and proactive stance toward change and continuous self-improvement" (Meyers, et al., p. 50). Ongoing learning and an expectation of positive growth throughout one's career ignites feelings of purpose and passion for one's work. Passion for work and a certainty that one's work has purpose and meaning are other elements that fill the deep well that ensures excellent practice.

In a far-reaching review of the research, Youssef-Morgan & Luthans (2015) clarify the positive relationship between psychological capital and well-being. The authors explain that the positive correlation is related to several elements, including the fact that fulfillment in significant life areas can lead to improved well-being. This additive and interactive relationship creates the "virtuous cycles" described in a previous chapter. In addition, psychological capital can facilitate awareness and retention of positive experiences, and therefore ensure a long-lasting impact on well-being.

Psychological capital increases evaluations of available personal resources, mitigates against the prevailing negativity bias, and reduces the likelihood of "hedonic adaptation" (Youssef-Morgan & Luthans, 2015). Hedonic adaptation refers to a tendency for human emotion to quickly return to a baseline level of happiness shortly after spikes in emotion caused by significantly positive or negative life events (Quoidbach & Dunn, 2013). However, merely abstaining from a favorite activity for a time as short as one week can reduce hedonic adaptation. It can be prevented simply by increasing diversity of experience. Working on a variety of life goals can help defend against the development of hedonic adaptation and sustain well-being (Youssef-Morgan & Luthans, 2015).

Replenishing the Well

The feelings of hope and efficacy associated with psychological capital encourage exceptional capabilities and outcomes in individuals. Resilience and optimism promote positive appraisals of circumstances and predictions of success (Youssef-Morgan & Luthans, 2015). It is easy to see how psychological capital is related to satisfied and well-performing practitioners, and consequently, we can understand how to increase psychological capital to replenish the deep well that promotes life enrichment and professional excellence. Psychological capital can be developed through education, intervention, and practice (Meyers, et al., 2015). Both strengths-based and deficiencies-based interventions can increase psychological capital, but greater increases in hope have been found with strengths-based interventions (Meyers, et al., 2015).

A logical place for this type of learning to take place is in the context of a mentoring relationship, clinical supervision, or a peer consultation group. It has been my experience that supervision hours often get taken up by discussions of "problem clients" or perceived therapeutic errors. A constant focus on the negative aspects of professional work will undermine resiliency and could be a contributing factor in professional burnout – it is equally important to elaborate on what is going well. Therefore, focusing on professional strengths is recommended as a starting point for building psychological capital. This positive focus is also essential when talking with friends and family about work. Due to the prevalent negativity bias, people tend to complain; constant complaining will erode well-being. Be as positive as possible about your work and you will notice more positive aspects of it.

Helping Professionals take note: Make sure that you focus in supervision or peer consultation on what you have done well. Celebrate your successes before you move on to talk about perceived weaknesses.

Job satisfaction is another element that replenishes the well. A special type of job satisfaction called "compassion satisfaction" applies to therapists because it highlights the powerful experience of emotional engagement necessary for successful therapeutic work (Figley & Ludick, 2017). Compassion satisfaction refers to the sense of fulfillment or pleasure that therapists feel when they have done their job well, such as the feelings of satisfaction derived from helping others. Being able to access these feelings of satisfaction has a protective effect against the development of secondary traumatic stress. The protective effect of job satisfaction is rooted in emotion and is separate from post-traumatic growth, which involves finding and developing meaning. Positive emotions can help focus attention and allow for the positive reframing of negative events, further promoting compassion satisfaction (Samios, Abel, & Rodzik, 2013).

Increasing one's positive emotions more generally is another way to increase psychological capital (Youssef-Morgan & Luthans, 2015). As was demonstrated in previous chapters, increasing positive emotions is one aspect of living an enriched life. It is possible to increase positive emotions through focusing on gratitude, listing "what went well today, and why," and writing about becoming one's best possible professional self (Hanson & Hanson, 2018; Seligman, 2011). Using signature strengths and savoring positive memories are also ways to increase positive emotions and replenish the well. Positive emotions are generated and maintained through regular physical exercise, which has proven anti-depressant effects (Garcia, et al., 2012; Hogan, et al., 2013; Sharma, Madaan, & Petty, 2006).

Living an enriched life fills the deep well with compassion that can make people more empathetic community members and allow for greater openness to helping others in meaningful ways. Sensuality and movement are the physical foundations for the deep well of life enrichment that helps boost one's quality of life far above the norm. Sensual experiences evoke beauty and positive emotions which contribute to the deep well of positivity, understanding, and compassion that characterizes an enriched life. In addition, experiencing positive emotions such as joy, contentment, pride and, especially awe has been shown to boost immune functioning by reducing levels of pro-inflammatory proteins (Hanson & Hanson, 2018; Stellar, et al., 2015). Positive emotions are not only enriching to the mind, they are enriching for the body as well. I often ask clients to create an image of what inspires awe in them; this way they have a concrete and powerful reminder of what can be a relatively rare occurrence. Plate 11 contains an example of a collage created by a client who wanted to remember the awe-inspiring effects of seeing the starry night sky on a camping trip to Yosemite. The image continued to generate feelings of wonder long after the experience was over.

In addition, because work is essential to our lives and influential to our sense of identity, having a solid sense of meaning and a related purpose in work are essential to living an enriched life. Meaning and purpose are additional elements that help refill the deep well of psychological resources supporting the excellent therapist. When job characteristics, personality traits, and professional motivation all work together, Helping Professionals experience meaningfulness. Indeed, the ability to engage in meaning-making is one of the things that portends the development of psychological growth.

Wide Margins

One way that I have encouraged people that I counsel to live an enriched life is to live with "wide margins." In order to live with wide margins, we first have to understand why they matter. In our fast-paced society we are constantly encouraged to do more and live without margins. Living without margins can cause anxiety, just like driving on a narrow road without a shoulder. When I describe living with wide margins, I mean that I intentionally leave more time than I think I will need between activities. I do not schedule the end of one meeting right up against the start of another. I allow at least a half an hour of downtime between finishing night activities and going to bed. I allow myself at least twice as much time as I need to get from one place to the next. For instance, I work between an outpatient office and a hospital setting. It is possible to travel door-to-door in 13 minutes if I rush, but I schedule myself 30 minutes between work places. This extra time gives me leeway to drive the speed limit, pause thoughtfully at the stop signs, and enjoy the beautiful views. It allows me time to stop and speak to the people who greet me in one location or the other. I can enrich my life every day with meaningful encounters, beautiful scenery, and mindful pauses. We have more time than we think we do to accomplish what is necessary. We do not have to hurry; our lives are enriched by a slower pace (Honoré, 2004; Sunim, 2017).

I once heard a mindfulness meditation teacher tell his students to say to themselves prior to doing any task, "I have time" and notice the effects on the mind and body. When people tell themselves that they have time, they take a deep breath, relax, and allow themselves to take their time to mindfully go about whatever it is they need to do. When prefaced with this short phrase, the activity is inevitably completed more calmly and enjoyably. Deep breathing activates the parasympathetic branch of the autonomic nervous system and initiates recovery after a stress response.

In case of an emergency, the stress response is meant to activate the sympathetic nervous system and the fight-or-flight response. After the emergency is over, the parasympathetic nervous system facilitates return of the body to a baseline, non-stressed state (Bracha, 2004). However, when people rush through their days, time pressure causes chronic activation of the stress response and the sympathetic nervous system. There is no opportunity for parasympathetic recovery. Living under chronic time pressure or other sources of stress is associated with many negative conditions such as obesity, heart disease, and depression (Kakiashvili, Leszek, & Rutkowski, 2013).

On the contrary, living life with wide margins means that leisure time is worked into each daily interaction: from stopping at the coffee shop in the morning to making the evening meal. Intentional pauses lead to increased enjoyment and greater physical relaxation. Taking time to smell the roses is associated with both physical and psychological well-being. In fact, one study literally showed increases in parasympathetic nervous system activation and decreases in self-rated stress when people paused to inhale the aroma of fresh roses (Igarashi, Song, Ikei, Ohira, & Miyazaki, 2014).

Pausing during the day provides time for self-reflection, which is impossible if people are rushed and busy. Rushing promotes a superficial glance or a cursory read, while taking time to really think or deeply ponder an idea requires time. We are rewarded for taking our time by a richer understanding of whatever concept caught our attention. In addition, when we slow down to reflect, we can experience our best selves rather than the harried and rushed self that easily becomes annoyed by the most minor inconvenience. Living with wide margins does not mean that everything is done slowly, just that everything has an appropriate tempo and we live in balance between efficiency and luxury (Honoré, 2004). Luxuriating in thought or deed is one element of living an enriched life.

Firm Boundaries

The diagram in Figure 11.1 demonstrates some of the boundaries that are necessary to support an enriched life. These include personal boundaries to ensure time for self-care and life enrichment, professional boundaries to reinforce appropriate work hours and an enriching work environment, and ethical boundaries with clients. As I have emphasized elsewhere in this book, in order to create and maintain firm boundaries of all types, people must realize that it is not selfish to focus on their own needs, but actually a form of self-preservation. When people constantly acquiesce to requests and violate their self-imposed restrictions around their personal time, requests can begin to feel like demands. Instead of giving with grace, overburdened people give grudgingly. Therefore, it is essential that therapists maintain good boundaries around personal time for enrichment so that the well is full and they have the capacity to giving willingly.

Compassionate people do not give of themselves without limits. They know themselves well – their strengths and limitations – and know what and how much they can give. They do say no to some requests so that they can wholeheartedly say yes to others (Brown, 2010). Saying no to some

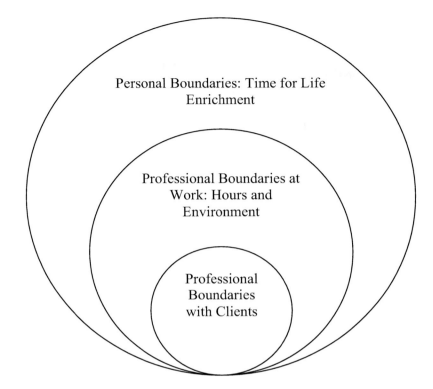

Figure 11.1 Diagram of Boundaries

requests means that therapists have time for all of the personal experiences that enrich their lives and fill the deep well of positive emotions that fuel a great career. Kind and empathic therapists have good boundaries.

Having clear professional boundaries is a hallmark of the successful Helping Professional (Figley & Ludick, 2017; Malinowski, 2014). The excellent therapist demonstrates the ability to set boundaries around work hours so that time and resources are available for life enrichment and self-care (Harrison & Westwood, 2009). In our fast-paced society where people love to complain about being too busy, it can be tempting to forgo physical or leisure activities to take on more work. However, when boundaries start to erode, repairs are often difficult and costly. The majority of people find it difficult to get back on track after allowing good habits and firm boundaries to lapse (McGonigal, 2013). Furthermore, lack of sleep and resulting cognitive impairment can cause poor decision-making and perhaps prompt harmful ethical violations in clinical practice.

Creating firm boundaries entails making schedules that highlight signature strengths and promote thriving in the work environment. Early career professionals are particularly susceptible to agreeing to every opportunity in the hope of making professional connections and cementing future work opportunities. However, many find that agreeing to many these commitments leaves them doing some amount of work that they do not enjoy and with too little time for leisure and enrichment. Perhaps it is better to begin with firm boundaries and trust that the right opportunities will occur in time. Another aspect of professional boundaries is making sure that you "own" your physical space by making it comfortable and pleasant. Adding pleasing paint colors and plants can boost well-being in the workplace.

Boundaries need to be flexible; they will change as personal and professional demands change. Therefore, self-reflection is necessary to ensure that boundaries are still supportive and not too restrictive. In Chapter 6, I recommended that a good time to review boundaries is at the beginning of each year. The New Year prompts reflection on goals and resolutions, so it is a good time to evaluate the occupational, social, familial, leisure, and spiritual aspects of life and whether more time or less time needs to be devoted to any of them. Beginning with personal boundaries and time for life enrichment, the LEM provides a starting place for this examination. Therapists can use the LEM to evaluate the physical, sensual, physical, emotional, intellectual, symbolic, and creative aspects of their lives and how they might be enhanced to provide greater life enrichment. Self-reflection is important for honoring what is in place as well as augmenting what is lacking.

Further exploring professional boundaries at work, it is worthwhile to spend time reflecting upon the work environment and relationships as well as the types of work being done. People tend to do the same thing at work year after year because change can feel threatening. Change is difficult because humans are hard-wired to seek safety. We tend to confuse comfort with safety, making it difficult to move on when a job is familiar, but no longer enlivening. I made this difficult discovery myself last year when I was reflecting on the various aspects of my professional life. It was surprising to realize that a teaching position that I had held for more than 15 years was no longer a source of joy. Had I not reviewed the status of my life in this way, I would still be doing a job that was familiar but not enlivening.

Finally, while performing their work, excellent clinicians are aware of ethical boundaries with clients that allow empathy to work within the therapeutic relationship without confusing client emotions with their own (Harrison & Westwood, 2009). The term "exquisite empathy" describes the way in which expert practitioners engage their clients with deep empathic accuracy, but with firm boundaries. These ethical boundaries are informed by ethical codes and flexibly enacted within the therapeutic relationship (Hinz, 2011). Even with clients, it is important to say no to requests that would erode personal time or cause too great a strain on resources. Therapists often have difficulty discussing fees and charging for their work. However, a fair fee is a necessary component to an excellent practice. Setting the fee partly denotes the importance of the work, and therapists are encouraged not to undersell themselves. Charging a fair rate helps people develop pride in their work and prevents them from becoming discouraged or resentful for having asked too little.

Dynamic Balance

Dynamic balance between LEM components is important because it encourages flexible responding. By "dynamic balance," I mean that activities from one side of any LEM level are performed in conjunction with those from another – they balance each other out. Working in dynamic balance feels good because it means that people are functioning optimally. Some examples include: Intellect and symbolism work together when a person comes out of a dream, a richly symbolic moment, and wants to decipher its meaning. If the person writes out a narrative of the dream or tries to relate it to the previous day's events, they are balancing the symbolism with an intellectual activity. Next, they might consider the meanings of universal and personal symbols (symbols from previous dreams), so they have moved back to symbolism. This back-and-forth activity facilitates discovery of the dream message and significance more thoroughly than either a purely intellectual or symbolic path.

In considering the next level, people evaluate the patterns and routines in their lives that soothe the emotions of everyday life. If commonly experienced emotions are anxiety or time pressure, routines help quiet the day-to-day worry. People might cook on the weekend (routine) to ease the daily anxiety (emotion) of what to prepare for dinner each night during the week. Finally, on the last level of the LEM, exercise feels good when it is balanced with sensation. After vigorous exercise, having a massage or taking a long shower is a balancing activity that enhances the gratifying feelings achieved from exercise. In addition, the dynamic balance here might involve balancing external rhythm and internal rhythm through music and movement.

Remember that it is not necessary to perform all of these activities in each day – a dynamic balance is always shifting and changing. Try to ensure that the majority of activities occur throughout the week and that none are neglected for any length of time. Moreover, if you have reflected on your life and decided that you need to add some enrichment, add it gradually instead of all at once. If too much change is undertaken at the same time it can be difficult to sustain the new habits and all of the new behaviors can be forsaken. It is better to add one new element at a time and linking a new behavior to an established one helps facilitate change (Duhigg, 2014).

Summary and Conclusions

Three essential elements of the enriched life are a deep well, wide margins, and firm boundaries. The deep well is full of psychological resources, physical vitality, and spiritual inspiration. It is the well that provides the reserves of energy and empathy necessary to conduct excellent clinical work. The well is replenished by increasing positive emotions, focusing on gratitude, and making sure to celebrate accomplishments. Having experiences with awe boosts physical and psychological well-being, refilling the well with positive emotion. To have wide margins means to have time built into the day for mindful practices, meaningful social interactions, and appreciation of beauty. Wide margins ensure time for intentional participation in self-reflection and creative practices, which ensure excellent self-care and clinical work. In order to create and maintain firm boundaries, therapists must be encouraged that it is not selfish to focus on their own needs. Firm boundaries preserve time for personal life enrichment, which further refreshes the deep well. In addition, having limits in place reminds therapists to take time to reflect upon their professional schedules, activities, and environments to ensure that they are enriching.

Living with all elements of the Life Enrichment Model in dynamic balance promotes optimal health. The movement and sensation level of the Life Enrichment Model emphasizes the physical vitality that is unique to each person and a foundation in sensual mindfulness to promote a stress-free life. These physical elements are fundamental for building strength and reducing stress; they establish the deep well of sustainable energy and empathy necessary for excellent work.

The next level of the LEM focuses on pattern/routine and emotions, allowing the formation of a life characterized by comfort and positive emotions. This level replenishes the deep well of psychological capital: hope, self-efficacy, resilience, and optimism. It helps cultivate empathy for self and others that enlivens one's personal life and professional practice. Activities on this level also reinforce the stable boundaries necessary to maintain a focus on personal life enrichment.

The intellect and symbolism level of the LEM focuses on the sophisticated cognitive and spiritual aspects of an enriched life. It helps people find meaning in their life and work and embrace activities that are personally and universally meaningful. A curious mind is enhanced by wide margins that ensure time for contemplation and curiosity, learning and living. Obtaining knowledge and having confidence in professional skills and abilities also fill the deep well that feeds an excellent clinical practice.

Finally, creativity is a broadly defined term that encompasses putting things or ideas together in ways that are novel and useful. These planned or serendipitous combinations enrich people's lives by encouraging flow experiences. It is through flow and creativity that people are in touch with their best possible selves. In addition, sharing creative experiences permits people to make deep connections with their highest expression of self, with others, and to connect with their higher power. All three types of connections occur most readily in the presence of wide margins, and all replenish the well of deep being or the deep well of being that supports an exceptionally enriched life.

The Life Enrichment Model was introduced as a structure to conceive and create an enriched and optimally healthy life. The consequences of life enrichment become the necessary conditions of it: a deep well, wide margins, and firm boundaries. Each component of this model provides essential experiences that replenish the deep and sustaining well, grant wide margins, and reinforce firm boundaries. These conditions then allow for intentional action within the LEM to provide even greater enrichment.

Art Reflections on an Enriched Life

1. Create an image that inspires you to remember to live with wide margins.
2. Make a collage of the things that "replenish your well" as a reminder that this well refreshes your personal and professional life.
3. Using the diagram in Figure 11.1 as a template, create a diagram of the boundaries in your personal and work life. Are there areas that need to be reinforced or loosened?

Questions for Self-Reflection

1. Choose a task you often rush through and go about it more slowly. What did you notice? How did it feel?
2. Is there any way that you could make your work space more personal, comfortable, or inviting? Add elements that would support a new view and feeling.
3. Take out the Life Enrichment Circle that you completed after reading the first chapter. How does it look to you now? Do you have a different perspective on what you would like the circle to look like?

References

Aftel, M. (2014). *Fragrant: The secret life of scent*. New York, NY: Riverhead books.
Alexander, B. (2010). Addiction: The view from Rat Park. Available at: www.brucek alexander.com/articles-speeches/rat-park/148-addiction-the-view-from-rat-park.
Alter, A. (2014). *Drunk tank pink: And other unexpected forces that shape how we think, feel, and behave*. New York, NY: Penguin Books.
American Psychological Association. (2017). *Stress in America: The state of our nation. Stress in America ™ Survey*. Washington DC: Author.
Andrade, J. (2010). What does doodling do? *Applied Cognitive Psychology*, 24(1), 100–106.
Arnheim, R. (1966). *Toward a psychology of art: Collected essays*. Berkeley and Los Angeles, CA: University of California Press.
Ashforth, B. E., Kreiner, G. E., & Fugate, M. (2000). All in a day's work: Boundaries and micro role transitions. *The Academy of Management Review*, 25(3), 472–491.
Ashokan, A., Hegde, A., & Mitra, R. (2016). Short-term environmental enrichment is sufficient to counter stress-induced anxiety and associated structural and molecular plasticity in basolateral amygdala. *Psychoneuroendocrinology*, 6(9), 189–196.
Babouchkina, A., & Robbins, S. J. (2015). Reducing negative mood through mandala creation: A randomized controlled trial. *Art Therapy: Journal of the American Art Therapy Association*, 32(1), 34–39.
Bagheri-Nesami, M., Espahbodi, F., Nikkhah, A., Shorofi, S., & Charati, J. (2014). The effects of lavender aromatherapy on pain following needle insertion into a fistula in hemodialysis patients. *Complementary Therapies in Clinical Practice*, 20(1), 1–4.
Bak, T. H., Nissan, J. J., Allerhand, M. M., & Deary, I. J. (2014). Does bilingualism influence cognitive aging? *Annals of Neurology*, 75(6), 959–963.
Barnard, L. K., & Curry, J. F. (2011). Self-compassion: Conceptualizations, correlates, & interventions. *Review of General Psychology*, 15(4), 289–303.
Barry, L. (2014). *Syllabus: Notes from an accidental professor*. Montreal, Canada: Drawn and Quarterly Publishers.
Bartoskova, L. (2015). Research into post-traumatic growth in therapists: A critical literature review. *Counselling Psychology Review*, 30(3), 57–68.

References

Bechdel, A. (2013). *Are you my mother: A comic drama*. New York, NY: Mariner Books.

Bernardi, L., Porta, C., & Sleight, P. (2006). Cardiovascular, cerebrovascular, and respiratory changes induced by different types of music in musicians and non-musicians: The importance of silence. *Heart*, 92(4), 445–452.

Bilodeau, C., Savard, R. & Lecomte, C. (2012). Trainee shame-proneness and the supervisory process. *The Journal for Counselor Preparation and Supervision*, 4(1), 37–48. Available at: http://repository.wcsu.edu/jcps/vol4/iss1/3

Bowen, D. H., Greene, J. P., & Kisida, B. (2014). Learning to think critically: A visual art experiment. *Educational Researcher*, 43(1), 37–44.

Bowen, M. T., & Neumann, I. D. (2017). Rebalancing the addicted brain: Oxytocin interference with the neural substrates of addiction. *Trends in Neurosciences*, 40(12), 691–708.

Bracha, S. (2004). Freeze, flight, fight, fright, faint: Adaptationist perspectives on the acute stress response spectrum. *CNS Spectrums*, 9(9), 679–85.

Bressler, S. L., & Menon, V. (2010). Large-scale brain networks in cognition: Emerging methods and principles. *Trends in Cognitive Sciences*, 14(6), 277–290.

Breus, M. (2006). *Good night: The sleep doctor's 4-week program to better sleep and better health*. New York, NY: Dutton.

Brown, B. (2010). *The gifts of imperfection: Let go of who you think you're supposed to be and embrace who you are*. Center City, MN: Hazelden.

Brown, Stuart. (2009). *Play: How it shapes the brain, opens the imagination, and invigorates the soul*. New York, NY: Avery/Penguin Group.

Brown, Sunni. (2015). *The doodle revolution: Unlock the power to think differently*. New York, NY: Portfolio.

Brown Taylor, B. (2009). *An altar in the world: A geography of faith*. New York, NY: Harper Collins.

Burns, D. D. (2008). *Feeling good: The new mood therapy*. New York, NY: Harper.

Bush, A. D. (2015). *Simple self-care for therapists: Restorative practices to weave through your workday*. New York, NY: Norton.

Caeyenberghs, K., & Leemans, A. (2014). Hemispheric lateralization of topological organization in structural brain networks. *Human Brain Mapping*, 35(9), 4944–4957.

Campbell, J. (1991). *The power of myth*. New York, NY: Anchor Books.

Canfield, J. (2005). Secondary traumatization, burnout, and vicarious traumatization: A review of the literature as it relates to therapists who treat trauma. *Smith College Studies in Social Work*, 75(2), 81–101.

Caspersen, C. J., Powell, K. E., & Christenson, G. M. (1985). Physical activity, exercise, and physical fitness: Definitions and distinctions for health-related research. *Public Health Reports*, 100(2), 126–131.

Cederström, C. & Spicer, A. (2015). *The wellness syndrome*. Cambridge, UK: Polity Books.

Chatterjee, A. (2015). The neuropsychology of visual art. In J. P. Huston, M. Nadal, F. Mora, L. F. Agnati, C. J. Cela-Conde, J. P. Huston, . . . C. J. Cela-Conde (Eds.), *Art, aesthetics and the brain* (pp. 341–356). London, UK: Oxford University Press.

Chen, M., Fang, S., & Fang, L. (2015). The effects of aromatherapy in relieving symptoms related to job stress among nurses. *International Journal of Nursing Practice*, 21(1), 87–93.

Chozen Bays, J. (2009). *Mindful eating: A guide to rediscovering a healthy and joyful relationship with food*. Boston, MA: Shambhala.

References

Coffeng, J. K., van Sluijs, E. M., Hendriksen, I. M., van Mechelen, W., & Boot, C. L. (2015). Physical activity and relaxation during and after work are independently associated with the need for recovery. *Journal of Physical Activity & Health*, 12(1), 109–115.

Collier, A. F. (2011). *Using textile arts and handcrafts in therapy with women: Weaving lives back together*. London, UK: Jessica Kingsley Publishers.

Connaughton, J., Patman, S., & Pardoe, C. (2014). Are there associations among physical activity, fatigue, sleep quality and pain in people with mental illness? A pilot study. *Journal of Psychiatric and Mental Health Nursing*, 21(8), 738–745.

Coolridge, S. T. (1853). *Works: Prose and verse complete*. Philadelphia, PA: Crissy & Markley.

Csikszentmihalyi, M. (2008). *Flow: The psychology of optimal experience*. New York, NY: Harper.

Curry, N. A. & Kasser, T. (2005). Can coloring mandalas reduce anxiety? *Art Therapy: Journal of the American Art Therapy Association*, 22(2), 81–85.

Dawkins, S., Martin, A., Scott, J., & Sanderson, K. (2013). Building on the positives: A psychometric review and critical analysis of the construct of Psychological Capital. *Journal of Occupational and Organizational Psychology*, 86(3), 348–370.

Deehan, G. J., Palmatier, M. I., Cain, M. E., & Kiefer, S. W. (2011). Differential rearing conditions and alcohol-preferring rats: Consumption of and operant responding for ethanol. *Behavioral Neuroscience*, 125(2), 184–193.

de Montaigne, M. (1999). The Essays. In C. B. Guignon (Ed.), *The good life: Reading in philosophy* (pp. 183–198). Indianapolis, IN: Hackett Publishing. (Original work published 1580).

De Oliveira, I. R., Seixas, C., Osório, F. L., Crippa, J. S., De Abreu, J. N., Menezes, I. G., & . . . Wenzel, A. (2015). Evaluation of the psychometric properties of the cognitive distortions questionnaire (CD-quest) in a sample of undergraduate students. *Innovations in Clinical Neuroscience*, 12(7–8), 20–27. Retrieved from: http://innovations cns.com/.

Dijkstra, K., Pieterse, M. E., & Pruyn, A. (2008). Stress-reducing effects of indoor plants in the built healthcare environment: The mediating role of perceived attractiveness. *Preventive Medicine*, 47(3), 279–283.

Dobek, C. E., Beynon, M. E., Bosma, R. L., & Stroman, P. W. (2014). Music modulation of pain perception and pain-related activity in the brain, brain stem, and spinal cord: A functional magnetic resonance imaging study. *The Journal of Pain*, 15(10), 1057–1068.

Duckworth, A. (2016). *Grit: The power of passion and perseverance*. New York, NY: Scribner.

Duhigg, C. (2014). *The power of habit: Why we do what we do in life and business*. New York, NY: Random House.

Edelkott, N., Engstrom, D. W., Hernandez-Wolfe, P., & Gangsei, D. (2016). Vicarious resilience: Complexities and variations. *American Journal of Orthopsychiatry*, 86(6), 713–724.

Ekman, P. (2007). *Emotions revealed: Recognizing faces and feelings to improve communication and emotional life* (2nd ed.). New York, NY: Holt Paperbacks.

Elavsky, S. (2010). Longitudinal examination of the exercise and self-esteem model in middle-aged women. *Journal of Sport & Exercise Psychology*, 32(6), 862–880.

Eliot, T. S. (1964). *Selected Essays of T.S. Eliot*. (New edition). New York, NY: Harcourt, Brace & World.

Emmons, R. A., & McCullough, M. E. (2003). Counting blessings versus burdens: An experimental investigation of gratitude and subjective well-being in daily life. *Journal of Personality and Social Psychology, 84*(2), 377–389.

Feldman Barrett, L. (2017). *How emotions are made: The secret life of the brain.* New York, NY: Houghton Mifflin Harcourt.

Ferrucci, P. (2009). *Beauty and soul: The extraordinary power of everyday beauty to heal your life.* New York, NY: Tarcher.

Figley, C. R., & Ludick, M. (2017). Secondary traumatization and compassion fatigue. In S. N. Gold (Ed.), *APA handbook of trauma psychology: Foundations in knowledge* (pp. 573–593). Washington, DC: American Psychological Association.

Fincher, S. F. (2000). *Coloring mandalas: For insight, healing and self-expression.* Boston, MA: Shambhala.

Fischer, E. (1959). *The necessity of art.* New York, NY: Penguin Books.

Fishel, A. K. (2015). *Home for dinner: Mixing food, fun, and conversation for a happier family and healthier kids.* San Francisco, CA: American Management Association.

Flausino, N. H., Da Silva Prado, J. M., De Queiroz, S. S., Tufik, S., & De Mello, M. T. (2012). Physical exercise performed before bedtime improves the sleep pattern of healthy young good sleepers. *Psychophysiology, 49*(2), 186–192.

Forgeard, M. C., Mecklenburg, A. C., Lacasse, J. J., & Jayawickreme, E. (2014). Bringing the whole universe to order: Creativity, healing, and posttraumatic growth. In J. C. Kaufman (Ed.), *Creativity and mental illness* (pp. 321–342). New York, NY: Cambridge University Press.

Forkosh, J., & Drake, J. E. (2017). Coloring versus drawing: Effects of cognitive demand on mood repair, flow, and enjoyment. *Art Therapy: Journal of the American Art Therapy Association, 34*(2), 75–82.

Forrer, K. (2015). Synchronicity: Did Jung have it right? *International Journal of Dream Research, 8*(2), 152–163.

Fox, M. (2002). *Illuminations of Hildegard of Bingen* (2nd ed.). Rochester, VT: Bear & Company.

Fredrickson, B. L. (2001). The role of positive emotions in positive psychology: The broaden-and-build theory of positive emotions. *American Psychologist, 56*(3), 218–226.

Frederiksen, K. S., Verdelho, A., Madureira, S., Bäzner, H., O'Brien, J. T., Fazekas, F., & ... Waldemar, G. (2015). Physical activity in the elderly is associated with improved executive function and processing speed: The LADIS study. *International Journal of Geriatric Psychiatry, 30*(7), 744–750.

Galaj, E., Manuszak, M., & Ranaldi, R. (2016). Environmental enrichment as a potential intervention for heroin seeking. *Drug and Alcohol Dependence, 16*(3), 195–201.

Galán, I., Meseguer, C. M., Herruzo, R., & Rodríguez-Artalejo, F. (2010). Self-rated health according to amount, intensity and duration of leisure time physical activity. *Preventive Medicine: An International Journal Devoted to Practice And Theory, 51*(5), 378–383.

Garcia, D., Archer, T., Moradi, S., & Andersson-Arntén, A. (2012). Exercise frequency, high activation, positive affect, and psychological wellbeing: Beyond age, gender, and occupation. *Psychology, 3*(4), 328–336.

Garcia, R. L., & Hand, C. J. (2016). Analgesic effects of self-chosen music type on cold pressor-induced pain: Motivating vs. relaxing music. *Psychology of Music, 44*(5), 967–983.

Gentzler, A. L., Palmer, C. A., & Ramsey, M. A. (2016). Savoring with intent: Investigating types of and motives for responses to positive events. *Journal of Happiness Studies, 17*(3), 937–958.

Gibson, D. (2017, November). A visual conversation with trauma: Using a visual journal to combat vicarious trauma. Paper presented at the 48th annual American Art Therapy Association Conference, Albuquerque, NM.

Gilbert, D. T., Pinel, E. C., Wilson, T. D., Blumberg, S. J., & Wheatley, T. P. (1998). Immune neglect: A source of durability bias in affective forecasting. *Journal of Personality and Social Psychology, 75*(3), 617–638.

Ginot, E. (2012). Self-narratives and dysregulated affective states: The neuropsychological links between self-narratives, attachment, affect, and cognition. *Psychoanalytic Psychology, 29*(1), 59–80.

Goleman, D. (2005). *Emotional intelligence: Why it can matter more than IQ*. New York, NY: Bantam.

Grandin, T., & Panek, R. (2013). *The autistic brain: Helping different kinds of minds succeed*. New York, NY: Houghton Mifflin.

Greenspan, M. (2003). *Healing through the dark emotions: The wisdom of grief, fear, and despair*. Boston, MA: Shambhala.

Gross, J. J. (2014). *Handbook of emotion regulation* (2nd ed.). New York, NY: Guilford.

Haar, J. M., Russo, M., Suñe, A., & Ollier-Malaterre, A. (2014). Outcomes of work–life balance on job satisfaction, life satisfaction and mental health: A study across seven cultures. *Journal of Vocational Behavior, 85*(3), 361–373.

Hall, K. (2012). *Zentangle untangled: Inspiration, and prompts for meditative drawing*. Cincinnati, OH: North Light Books.

Hanson, R. (2017, May). H.E.A.L. your creativity and grow your resources. Createfest: The second annual online creativity festival for mental health professionals.

Hanson, R. & Hanson, F. (2018). *Resilient: How to grow an unshakable core of calm, strength, and happiness*. New York, NY: Harmony Books.

Harris, P. R. (2011). Self-affirmation and the self-regulation of health behavior change. *Self and Identity, 10*(3), 304–314.

Harrison, R. L., & Westwood, M. J. (2009). Preventing vicarious traumatization of mental health therapists: Identifying protective practices. *Psychotherapy: Theory, Research, Practice, Training, 46*(2), 203–219.

Harter, S. L. (2007). Visual art making for therapist growth and self-care. *Journal of Constructivist Psychology, 20*(2), 167–182.

Hartescu, I., Morgan, K., & Stevinson, C. D. (2015). Increased physical activity improves sleep and mood outcomes in inactive people with insomnia: A randomized controlled trial. *Journal of Sleep Research, 24*(5), 526–534.

Henderson, P., Rosen, D., & Mascaro, N. (2007). Empirical study on the healing nature of mandalas. *Psychology of Aesthetics, Creativity, and the Arts, 1*(3), 148–154.

Hinz, L. D. (2006). *Drawing from within: Using art to treat eating disorders*. London, UK: Jessica Kingsley Publishers.

Hinz, L. D. (2009). *Expressive Therapies Continuum: A framework for using art in therapy*. New York, NY: Routledge.

Hinz, L. D. (2011). Embracing excellence: A positive approach to ethical decision making. *Art Therapy: Journal of the American Art Therapy Association, 28*(4), 1–4.

Hoang, T. D., Reis, J., Zhu, N., Jacobs, D. J., Launer, L. J., Whitmer, R. A., & . . . Yaffe, K. (2016). Effect of early adult patterns of physical activity and television viewing on midlife cognitive function. *JAMA Psychiatry*, 73(1), 73–79.

Hogan, C. L., Mata, J., & Carstensen, L. L. (2013). Exercise holds immediate benefits for affect and cognition in younger and older adults. *Psychology and Aging*, 28(2), 587–594.

Hollis, J. (2008). *Why good people do bad things: Understanding our darker selves*. New York, NY: Avery Press.

Holton, M. K., Barry, A. E., & Chaney, J. D. (2016). Employee stress management: An examination of adaptive and maladaptive coping strategies on employee health. *Work: Journal of Prevention, Assessment & Rehabilitation*, 53(2), 299–305.

Honoré, C. (2004). *In praise of slowness: Challenging the cult of speed*. New York, NY: Harper Collins.

Howard, S., & Hughes, B. M. (2008). Expectancies, not aroma, explain impact of lavender aromatherapy on psychophysiological indices of relaxation in young healthy women. *British Journal of Health Psychology*, 13(4), 603–617.

Hsieh, C., Kong, J., Kirsch, I., Edwards, R. R., Jensen, K. B., Kaptchuk, T. J., & Gollub, R. L. (2014). Well-loved music robustly relieves pain: A randomized, controlled trial. *Plos ONE*, 9(9), 1–8.

Hur, M., Song, J., Lee, J., & Lee, M. S. (2014). Aromatherapy for stress reduction in healthy adults: A systematic review and meta-analysis of randomized clinical trials. *Maturitas*, 79(4), 362–369.

Hurley, D. B., & Kwon, P. (2012). Results of a study to increase savoring the moment: Differential impact on positive and negative outcomes. *Journal of Happiness Studies*, 13(4), 579–588.

Hüttermann, S., & Memmert, D. (2012). Moderate movement, more vision: Effects of physical exercise on inattentional blindness. *Perception*, 41(8), 963–975.

Hwang, E., & Shin, S. (2015). The effects of aromatherapy on sleep improvement: A systematic literature review and meta-analysis. *The Journal of Alternative and Complementary Medicine*, 21(2), 61–68.

Igarashi, M., Song, C., Ikei, H., Ohira, T., & Miyazaki, Y. (2014). Effect of olfactory stimulation by fresh rose flowers on autonomic nervous activity. *The Journal of Alternative and Complementary Medicine*, 20(9), 727–731.

Jackowska, M., Brown, J., Ronaldson, A., & Steptoe, A. (2016). The impact of a brief gratitude intervention on subjective well-being, biology and sleep. *Journal of Health Psychology*, 21(10), 2207–2217.

Jacobi, J. (1961). *Psychological reflections: An anthology of the writings of C. G. Jung*. New York, NY: Harper.

Jha, T., Pawar, A., Jha, K. M., Monga, M., Mondal, S., & Gandhi, A. (2015). The effect of Indian classical music on migraine episodes in young females of age group 18 to 23 years. *Music and Medicine*, 7(4), 24–31. Retrieved from: http://mmd.iammonline.com/index.php/musmed/article/view/431/0.

Jose, P. E., Lim, B. T., & Bryant, F. B. (2012). Does savoring increase happiness? A daily diary study. *The Journal of Positive Psychology*, 7(3), 176–187.

Joseph, S., Murphy, D., & Regel, S. (2012). An affective-cognitive processing model of post-traumatic growth. *Clinical Psychology and Psychotherapy*, 19(4), 316–325.

Joyce Carol Oats Writes Memoir of Grief (2011). Retrieved from: www.cbsnews.com/news/joyce-carol-oates-writes-memoir-of-grief/.

Kagge, E. (2017). *Silence: In the age of noise*. New York, NY: Viking Press.
Kagin, S. L., & Lusebrink, V. B. (1978). The expressive therapies continuum. *Art Psychotherapy*, 5(4), 171–180.
Kahneman, D. (2011). *Thinking, fast and slow*. New York, NY: Farrar, Straus and Giroux.
Kakiashvili, T., Leszek, J., & Rutkowski, K. (2013). The medical perspective on burnout. *International Journal of Occupational Medicine and Environmental Health*, 26(3), 401–412.
Kaminsky, P. (2013). *Culinary intelligence: The art of eating healthy (and really well)*. New York, NY: Vintage.
Kavoor, A. R., Mitra, S., Mahintamani, T., & Chatterjee, S. S. (2015). Primary prevention of Alzheimer's disease in developing countries. *Clinical Psychopharmacology and Neuroscience*, 13(3), 327.
Keats, J. (1899). *The complete poetical works and letters of Keats: Cambridge edition*, (Edited by H. E.Scudder). Boston, MA: Houghton Mifflin.
Kelley, T. & Kelley, D. (2013). *Creative confidence: Unleashing the creative potential within us all*. New York, NY: Crown Books.
Kersten, A. & van der Vennet, R. (2010). The impact of anxious and calm emotional states on color usage in pre-drawn mandalas. *Art Therapy: Journal of the American Art Therapy Association*, 27(4), 184–189.
Kiecolt-Glaser, J. K., Graham, J. E., Malarkey, W. B., Porter, K., Lemeshow, S., & Glaser, R. (2008). Olfactory influences on mood and autonomic, endocrine, and immune function. *Psychoneuroendocrinology*, 33(3), 328–339.
Kim, J. (2015). Physical activity benefits creativity: Squeezing a ball for enhancing creativity. *Creativity Research Journal*, 27(4), 328–333.
Kim, S., & Ki, J. (2014). A case study on the effects of the creative art therapy with stretching and walking meditation—Focusing on the improvement of emotional expression and alleviation of somatisation symptoms in a neurasthenic adolescent. *The Arts in Psychotherapy*, 41(1), 71–78.
King, A. J. (2017). Using comics to communicate about health: An introduction to the symposium on visual narratives and graphic medicine. *Health Communication*, 32(5), 523–524.
Kinsbourne, M. (2011). Repetitive movements and arousal. In D. Fien (Ed.), *The neuropsychology of autism* (pp. 367–394). London, UK: Oxford University Press.
Kirste, I., Nicola, Z., Kronenberg, G., Walker, T. L., Liu, R. C., & Kempermann, G. (2015). Is silence golden? Effects of auditory stimuli and their absence on adult hippocampal neurogenesis. *Brain Structure and Function*, 220(2), 1221–1228.
Koch, S., Kunz, T., Lykou, S., & Cruz, R. (2014). Effects of dance movement therapy and dance on health-related psychological outcomes: A meta-analysis. *The Arts in Psychotherapy*, 41(1), 46–64.
Kohn, M., Belza, B., Petrescu-Prahova, M., & Miyawaki, C. E. (2016). Beyond strength: Participant perspectives on the benefits of an older adult exercise program. *Health Education & Behavior*, 43(3), 305–312.
Kondo, M. (2014). *The life-changing magic of tidying up*. New York, NY: Ten Speed Press.
Kopcsó, K., & Láng, A. (2017). Regulated divergence: Textual patterns, creativity and cognitive emotion regulation. *Creativity Research Journal*, 29(2), 218–223.
Kottler, J.A. (2017). *On being a therapist* (5th ed.). London, UK: Oxford University Press.

Kredlow, M. A., Capozzoli, M. C., Hearon, B. A., Calkins, A. W., & Otto, M. W. (2015). The effects of physical activity on sleep: A meta-analytic review. *Journal of Behavioral Medicine, 38*(3), 427–449.

L'Abate, L. (2016). Intimacy and sharing hurts. In G. R. Weeks, S. T. Fife, & C. M. Peterson (Eds.), *Techniques for the couple therapist: Essential interventions from the experts* (pp. 151–154). New York, NY: Routledge.

Lambert, N. M., Fincham, F. D., & Stillman, T. F. (2012). Gratitude and depressive symptoms: The role of positive reframing and positive emotion. *Cognition and Emotion, 26*(4), 615–633.

Lao, T. (1996). *Tao Teh King. Interpreted as nature and intelligence* (A. J. Baum, Trans.). Freemont, CA: Jain Publishing. (original work published 6th century B.C.E.)

Layous, K., Nelson, S. K., & Lyubomirsky, S. (2013). What is the optimal way to deliver a positive activity intervention? The case of writing about one's best possible selves. *Journal of Happiness Studies, 14*(2), 635–654.

Lehrer, J. (2012). *Imagine: How creativity works*. New York: Houghton Mifflin.

Lesiuk, T. (2008). The effect of preferred music listening on stress levels of air traffic controllers. *The Arts in Psychotherapy, 35*(1), 1–10.

Levitin, D. J. (2007). *This is your brain on music: The science of a human obsession*. New York, NY: Plume/Penguin.

Li, Q. (2018). *Forest bathing: How trees can help you find health and happiness*. New York, NY: Penguin Random House.

Lichtenfeld, S., Elliot, A. J., Maier, M. A., & Pekrun, R. (2012). Fertile green: Green facilitates creative performance. *Personality and Social Psychology Bulletin, 38*(6), 784–797.

Lillehei, A. S. & Halcon, L. L. (2014). A systematic review of the effect of inhaled essential oils on sleep. *Journal of Alternative and Complementary Medicine, 20*(6), 441–451.

Liu, D. Y., & Thompson, R. J. (2017). Selection and implementation of emotion regulation strategies in major depressive disorder: An integrative review. *Clinical Psychology Review, 57*, 183–194.

Lobel, T. (2014). *Sensation: The new science of physical intelligence*. New York, NY: Atria Books.

Lomas, T., Hefferon, K., & Ivtzan, I. (2014). *Applied positive psychology: Integrated positive practice*. London, UK: Sage Publications.

Longfellow, H. W. (1884). *The poetical works of Henry Wadsworth Longfellow*. Boston, MA: Houghton Mifflin and Company.

Louv, R. (2011). *The nature principle: Human restoration and the end of nature-deficit disorder*. Chapel Hill, NC: Algonquin Books.

Luken, M., & Sammons, A. (2016). Systematic review of mindfulness practice for reducing job burnout. *American Journal of Occupational Therapy, 70*(2), 1–10.

Lusebrink, V. B. (1990). *Imagery and visual expression in therapy*. New York: Plenum Press.

Lusebrink, V. B. (1991). A systems oriented approach to the expressive therapies: The Expressive Therapies Continuum. *The Arts in Psychotherapy, 18*(5), 395–403.

Lusebrink, V. B. (2004). Art therapy and the brain: An attempt to understand the underlying processes of art expression in therapy. *Art Therapy: Journal of the American Art Therapy Association, 21*(3), 125–135.

Lusebrink, V. B. (2010). Assessment and therapeutic application of the Expressive Therapies Continuum: Implications for brain structures and functions. *Art Therapy: Journal of the American Art Therapy Association, 27*(4), 168–177.

Lusebrink, V. B. (2014). Art therapy and neural basis of imagery: Another possible view. *Art Therapy: Journal of the American Art Therapy Association, 31*(2), 87–90.

Lytle, J., Mwatha, C., & Davis, K. K. (2014). Effect of lavender aromatherapy on vital signs and perceived quality of sleep in the intermediate care unit: A pilot study. *American Journal of Critical Care, 23*(1), 24–29.

McCormack, L., & Adams, E. L. (2016). Therapists, complex trauma, and the medical model: Making meaning of vicarious distress from complex trauma in the inpatient setting. *Traumatology, 22*(3), 192–202.

McGonigal, K. (2013). *The willpower instinct: How self-control works, why it matters, and what you can do to get more of it.* New York, NY: Avery.

MacLean, P. D. (1985). Evolutionary psychiatry and the triune brain. *Psychological Medicine, 15*(2), 219–221.

McNeill, D. P, Morrison, D. A., & Nouwen, H. J. M. (2006). *Compassion: A reflection on the Christian life* (rev. ed.). New York, NY: Image Books.

Malinowki, A. J. (2014). *Self-care for the mental health practitioner: The theory, research, and practice of preventing and addressing the occupational hazards of the profession.* London, UK: Jessica Kingsley Publishers.

Martela, F., & Steger, M. F. (2016). The three meanings of meaning in life: Distinguishing coherence, purpose, and significance. *The Journal of Positive Psychology, 11*(5), 531–545.

Mehta, R., & Zhu, R. (2009). Blue or red? Exploring the effect of color on cognitive task performances. *Science, 323*(5918), 1226–1229.

Meier, A., & Musick, K. (2014). Variation in associations between family dinners and adolescent well-being. *Journal of Marriage and Family, 76*(1), 13–23.

Merton, T. (1983). *No man is an island.* New York, NY: Houghton Mifflin.

Meyers, M. C., van Woerkom, M., de Reuver, R. M., Bakk, Z., & Oberski, D. L. (2015). Enhancing psychological capital and personal growth initiative: Working on strengths or deficiencies. *Journal of Counseling Psychology, 62*(1), 50–62.

Milton, J. (2016). *Areopagitica and other prose works.* Mineola, NY: Courier Dover Publications. (Original work published 1644).

Molino, M., Ghislieri, C., & Cortese, C. G. (2013). When work enriches family-life: The mediational role of professional development opportunities. *Journal of Workplace Learning, 25*(2), 98–113.

Montessori, M. (1967). *The absorbent mind.* New York, NY: Dell.

Morgan, J. P., MacDonald, R. R., & Pitts, S. E. (2015). 'Caught between a scream and a hug': Women's perspectives on music listening and interaction with teenagers in the family unit. *Psychology of Music, 43*(5), 611–626.

Mullenbach, M. & Skovholt, T. M. (2001). Burnout prevention and self-care strategies of expert practitioners. In T. M. Skovholt (Ed.), *The resilient practitioner: Burnout prevention and self-care strategies for counselors, therapists, teachers, and health care professionals* (pp. 163–186). Boston, MA: Allyn & Bacon.

Neff, K. D. (2003). Self-compassion: An alternative conceptualization of a healthy attitude toward oneself. *Self and Identity, 2*(2), 85–101.

Newell, J. M., Nelson-Gardell, D., & MacNeil, G. (2016). Clinician responses to client traumas: A chronological review of constructs and terminology. *Trauma, Violence, & Abuse*, 17(3), 306–313.

Newman, A., Ucbasaran, D., Zhu, F., & Hirst, G. (2014). Psychological capital: A review and synthesis. *Journal of Organizational Behavior*, 35(1), 120–138.

Nezlek, J. B., Newman, D. B., & Thrash, T. M. (2017). A daily diary study of relationships between feelings of gratitude and well-being. *The Journal of Positive Psychology*, 12(4), 323–332.

Niemiec, R. M. (2014). *Mindfulness and character strengths: A practical guide to flourishing*. Cambridge, MA: Hogrefe.

Norcross, J. C. & Guy, J. D. (2007). *Leaving it at the office: A guide to psychotherapist self-care*. New York, NY: Guilford.

O'Donohue, J. (2008). *To bless the space between us: A book of blessings*. New York, NY: Doubleday.

Osho. (2002). *Fear of intimacy*. [Kindle DX version]. Retrieved from Amazon.com.

Park, C. L., Currier, J. M., Harris, J. I., & Slattery, J. M. (2017). *Trauma, meaning, and spirituality: Translating research into clinical practice*. Washington, DC: American Psychological Association.

Penn, W. (1726). *A collection of the works of William Penn* (Vol. 1). London, UK: J. Sowle Publisher.

Piaget, J. (2000). Piaget's theory. In K. Lee (Ed.), *Childhood cognitive development: The essential readings* (pp. 33–47). Malden, MA: Blackwell Publishing.

Pickett, K., Kendrick, T., & Yardley, L. (2017). 'A forward movement into life': A qualitative study of how, why and when physical activity may benefit depression. *Mental Health and Physical Activity*, 12, 100–109.

Plante, T. G., Gustafson, C., Brecht, C., Imberi, J., & Sanchez, J. (2011). Exercising with an iPod, friend, or neither: Which is better for psychological benefits? *American Journal of Health Behavior*, 35(2), 199–208.

Plato. (1945). *The republic of Plato*. F. M. Cornford (Ed., Trans.). New York, NY: Oxford University Press (Original work published 380 BCE).

Powers, M. B., Asmundson, G. G., & Smits, J. J. (2015). Exercise for mood and anxiety disorders: The state-of-the science. *Cognitive Behaviour Therapy*, 44(4), 237–239.

Puig, A., Baggs, A., Mixon, K., Park, Y. M., Kim, B. Y., & Lee, S. M. (2012). Relationship between job burnout and personal wellness in mental health professionals. *Journal of Employment Counseling*, 49(3), 98–109.

Quiroga Murcia, C., Kreutz, G., Clift, S., & Bongard, S. (2010). Shall we dance? An exploration of the perceived benefits of dancing on well-being. *Arts & Health: An International Journal of Research, Policy and Practice*, 2(2), 149–163.

Quoidbach, J., & Dunn, E. W. (2013). Give it up: A strategy for combating hedonic adaptation. *Social Psychological and Personality Science*, 4(5), 563–568.

Ratey, J. J., & Hagerman, E. (2008). *Spark: The revolutionary new science of exercise and the brain*. New York, NY: Little, Brown, & Company.

Ratey, J. J., & Manning, R. (2015). *Go wild: Eat fat, run free, be social, and follow evolution's other rules for total health and well-being*. New York: Little, Brown, & Company.

Redstone, L. (2015). Mindfulness meditation and aromatherapy to reduce stress and anxiety. *Archives of Psychiatric Nursing*, 29(3), 192–193.

References

Rehfeld, K., Müller, P., Aye, N., Schmicker, M., Dordevic, M., Kaufmann, J., & . . . Müller, N. G. (2017). Dancing or fitness sport? The effects of two training programs on hippocampal plasticity and balance abilities in healthy seniors. *Frontiers in Human Neuroscience*, 11(305), 1–9.

Richards, R. (2014). A creative alchemy. In S. Moran, D. Cropley, & J. C. Kaufman, (Eds.), *The ethics of creativity* (pp. 119–136). New York, NY: Palgrave Macmillan.

Riley, K. E., & Park, C. L. (2015). How does yoga reduce stress? A systematic review of mechanisms of change and guide to future inquiry. *Health Psychology Review*, 9(3), 379–396.

Rogerson, M.D., Gottlieb, M.C., Handelsman, M.M, Knapp, S., & Younggren, J. (2011). Non-rational processes in ethical decision making. *American Psychologist*, 66(7), 614–623.

Rossner, M., & Meher, M. (2014). Emotions in ritual theories. In J. E. Stets, & J. H. Turner (Eds.), *Handbook of the sociology of emotions*, Vol. 2 (pp. 199–220). New York, NY: Springer.

Rozin, P., & Royzman, E. B. (2001). Negativity bias, negativity dominance, and contagion. *Personality and Social Psychology Review*, 5(4), 296–320.

Rudd, M., Vohs, K. D., & Aaker, J. (2012). Awe expands people's perception of time, alters decision making, and enhances well-being. *Psychological Science*, 23(10), 1130–1136.

Runco, M. A., & Jaeger, G. J. (2012). The standard definition of creativity. *Creativity Research Journal*, 24(1), 92–96.

Ruud, E. (2013). Can music serve as a "cultural immunogen"? An explorative study. *International Journal of Qualitative Studies on Health and Well-Being*, 1–12.

Sakuragi, S., & Sugiyama, Y. (2011). Effect of partition board color on mood and autonomic nervous function. *Perceptual and Motor Skills*, 113(3), 941–956.

Saint Irenaeus (180). *Against heresies* (Book IV, Chapter 20, p. 4). Retrieved from: http://ia802307.us.archive.org/7/items/SaintIrenaeusAgainstHeresiesComplete/Saint_Irenaeus_Against_Heresies_Complete.pdf

Salzano, A. T., Lindemann, E., & Tronsky, L. N. (2013). The effectiveness of a collaborative art-making task on reducing stress in hospice caregivers. *The Arts in Psychotherapy*, 40(1), 45–52.

Samios, C., Abel, L. M., & Rodzik, A. K. (2013). The protective role of compassion satisfaction for therapists who work with sexual violence survivors: An application of the broaden-and-build theory of positive emotions. *Anxiety, Stress & Coping: An International Journal*, 26(6), 610–623.

Sasannejad, P., Saeedi, M., Shoeibi, A., Gorji, A., Abbasi, M., & Foroughipour, M. (2012). Lavender essential oil in the treatment of migraine headache: A placebo-controlled clinical trial. *European Neurology*, 67(5), 288–291.

Scarapicchia, T. F., Amireault, S., Faulkner, G., & Sabiston, C. M. (2017). Social support and physical activity participation among healthy adults: A systematic review of prospective studies. *International Review of Sport and Exercise Psychology*, 10(1), 50–83.

Schmidt, K., Beck, R., Rivkin, W., & Diestel, S. (2016). Self-control demands at work and psychological strain: The moderating role of physical fitness. *International Journal of Stress Management*, 23(3), 255–275.

Schopenhauer, A. (1958). *The world as will and representation* (Vol. 2). (E. F. J. Payne, Trans.). New York, NY: Dover Publications. (Original work published 1859).

Schott, G. D. (2011). Doodling and the default network of the brain. *The Lancet*, 378(9797), 1133–1134.

Seligman, M. P. (2011). *Flourish: A visionary new understanding of happiness and wellbeing.* New York, NY: Free Press.

Sellaro, R., Hommel, B., Rossi Paccani, C., & Colzato, L. S. (2015). With peppermints you're not my prince: Aroma modulates self-other integration. *Attention, Perception, & Psychophysics*, 77(8), 2817–2825.

Seneca, L. A. (2016). *Seneca's letters from a stoic.* (R. M. Gummere, Trans.). Mineloa, NY: Dover Thrift Publications. (Original work published 65 A.D.)

Sened, H., Lavidor, M., Lazarus, G., Bar-Kalifa, E., Rafaeli, E., & Ickes, W. (2017). Empathic accuracy and relationship satisfaction: A meta-analytic review. *Journal of Family Psychology*, 31(6), 742–752.

Sharma, A., Madaan, V., & Petty, F. D. (2006). Exercise for mental health. *Primary Care Companion to the Journal of Clinical Psychiatry*, 8(2), 106. Retrieved from: http://europepmc.org/articles/PMC1470658

Silvia, P. J., Beaty, R. E., Nusbaum, E. C., Eddington, K. M., Levin-Aspenson, H., & Kwapil, T. R. (2014). Everyday creativity in daily life: An experience-sampling study of "little c" creativity. *Psychology of Aesthetics, Creativity, and the Arts*, 8(2), 183–188.

Singh, T., & Kashyap, N. (2015). Does doodling effect performance: Comparison across retrieval strategies. *Psychological Studies*, 60(1), 7–11.

Sis, P. (2011). *The conference of the birds.* New York, NY: Penguin Press.

Smith, J. L., & Bryant, F. B. (2016). The benefits of savoring life: Savoring as a moderator of the relationship between health and life satisfaction in older adults. *The International Journal of Aging & Human Development*, 84(1), 3–23.

Smith, L. (2016). *No fears, no excuses: What you need to do to have a great career.* New York, NY: Houghton, Mifflin, Harcourt.

Steele, W., & Kuban, C. (2012). Using drawing in short-term trauma resolution. In C. A. Malchiodi (Ed.), *Handbook of art therapy.* (2nd ed.). (pp. 162–174). New York, NY: Guilford Press.

Stellar, J. E., John-Henderson, N., Anderson, C. L., Gordon, A. M., McNeil, G. D., & Keltner, D. (2015). Positive affect and markers of inflammation: Discrete positive emotions predict lower levels of inflammatory cytokines. *Emotion*, 15(2), 129–133.

Stone, H., & Stone, S. (1993). *Embracing your inner critic: Turning self-criticism into a creative asset.* New York, NY: HarperOne.

Strahler, J., Doerr, J. M., Ditzen, B., Linnemann, A., Skoluda, N., & Nater, U. M. (2016). Physical activity buffers fatigue only under low chronic stress. *Stress: The International Journal on the Biology of Stress*, 19(5), 535–541.

Sunim, H. (2017). *The things you can see only when you slow down: how to be calm and mindful in a fast-paced world.* New York, NY: Penguin Books.

Tang, S. K., & Tse, M. M. (2014). Aromatherapy: Does it help to relieve pain, depression, anxiety, and stress in community-dwelling older persons? *Biomed Research International*, 2014, Article ID: 430195.

Tedeschi, R. G., & Calhoun, L. G. (1996). The Posttraumatic Growth Inventory: Measuring the positive legacy of trauma. *Journal of Traumatic Stress*, 9(3), 455–472.

Thayer, R. E. (2001). *Calm energy: How people regulate mood with food and exercise.* London, UK: Oxford University Press.

Thoreau, H. D. (2009). *The journal of Henry David Thoreau, 1837–1861*. D. Searls (Ed.). New York, NY: New York Review Books Classics. (Originally published in 1951).

Turgoose, D., & Maddox, L. (2017). Predictors of compassion fatigue in mental health professionals: A narrative review. *Traumatology, 23*(2), 172–185.

van der Vennet, R., & Serice, S. (2012). Can coloring mandalas reduce anxiety? A replication study. *Art Therapy: Journal of the American Art Therapy Association, 29*(2), 87–92.

Vartanian, O., & Skov, M. (2014). Neural correlates of viewing paintings: Evidence from a quantitative meta-analysis of functional magnetic resonance imaging data. *Brain and Cognition, 87*(1), 52–56.

Vessel, E. A., Starr, G. G., & Rubin, N. (2002). The brain on art: intense aesthetic experience activates the default mode network. *Frontiers in Human Neuroscience, 6* (66), 1–17.

Walker, M. (2017). *Why we sleep: Unlocking the power of sleep and dreams*. New York, NY: Scribner.

Whyte, D. (2016). *Consolations: The solace, nourishment and underlying meaning of everyday words*. Langley, WA: Many Rivers Press.

Wicks, R. J. (2007). *The resilient clinician*. London, UK: Oxford University Press.

Wilkinson, R. A., & Chilton, G. (2017). *Positive Art Therapy Theory and Practice: Integrating Positive Psychology with Art Therapy*. New York, NY: Routledge.

Wolpert, D. M., Diedrichsen, J., & Flanagan, J. R. (2011). Principles of sensorimotor learning. *Nature Reviews Neuroscience, 12*, 739–751.

Youssef-Morgan, C. M., & Luthans, F. (2015). Psychological capital and well-being. *Stress and Health: Journal of the International Society for the Investigation of Stress, 31*(3), 180–188.

Želeskov-Dorić, J., Hedrih, V., & Dorić, P. (2012). Relations of resilience and personal meaning with vicarious traumatization in psychotherapists. *International Journal of Psychotherapy, 16*(3), 44–55. Retrieved from: www.academia.edu/12135827.

Zhang, J., & Yen, S. T. (2015). Physical activity, gender difference, and depressive symptoms. *Health Services Research, 50*(5), 1550–1573.

Index

aerobic exercise 41, 43
Alexander, B. 13
altruism 6
American Psychological Association (APA) 12
antidepressant effects 41
anxiety 34, 44, 52
APA *see* American Psychological Association (APA)
aroma 28; almond 28; cinnamon 28; lavender 28, 29; lemon 28; peppermint 28, 29; as a complementary therapy 28; relaxing 29; sharing 29
art 85–86
art experience: through movement 41
artistic media 17
art therapist 2, 29
auditory sensation and silence 33–34
autism 72
autobiographical thought 86

blood pressure 34
books, illustrated 90
brainstorming 99
Brown, B. 57
Brown, S. 97
Buddhist concept 74

calm energy 43, 44
Campbell, J. 30, 89
carpal tunnel syndrome 31
Carstensen, L. L. 42
cause-and-effect thinking 71
classical music 34
cognitive process 83
colored flowers 33
coloring books 54
color spectrum 29
community supported agriculture (CSA) 32
compassion 5, 27; fatigue 4, 5; satisfaction 107
countertransference 6
creativity 21–22; and art reflection 103; and connection 99; and flow 96–97; increasing 99–102; and play 97–98; and psychological growth 98–99
critical thinking skills 85
Csikszentmihalyi, M. 95
Culinary Intelligence 32
cultural immunogen 68
curiosity/learning, at work 77

dance 45–46
decision making 67–68, 71
Default Mode Network (DMN) 35

depression 72
Direct Experience Network (DEN) 35
doodling 54
dreams 91
dynamic balance 24, 113–114

Eliot, T. S. 90
emotion 20–21, 41; and art reflection 69–70; and decision making 67–68; enrichment through 69; increasing positive 63–64; purpose of 62–63; regulation of 65–66; sharing 64–65; symbolic thinking 83
emotional fatigue 5
emotionally draining therapy 66
emotional signals 62
empathic accuracy 55
empathy 6; exquisite 55
enriched life: characters 27
enriched life practice 105; art reflections on 115; a deep well 106–107; dynamic balance 113–114; firm boundaries 110–113; replenishing the well 107–108; wide margins 109–110
environmental enrichment 30
ETC *see* Expressive Therapies Continuum (ETC)
exercise, benefits of 40
Expressive Therapies Continuum (ETC) 17
exquisite empathy 55

fast thinking 83
fatigue 43–44
fight-or-flight response 109
firm boundaries 110–113
first time–last time experience 36
Fischer, E. 85
frankincense 28
Functional Magnetic Resonance Imaging (fMRI) 35

Gestalt psychology 51
Gibson, D. 66
Gifts of Imperfection, The 57
Ginot, E. 72

golden pathos (plant) 30
Grit 78–79

habituation 36
Hanson, R. 101
healthy people 14
hedonic adaptation 106
heuristics 67
Hogan, C. L. 42
holistic health 2
houseplant 30
hug 31
hunger, types of 32

Imagine: How Creativity Works 100
immune function 34
intellect component, LEM: and Art Reflection 80; curiosity/learning at work 77; developing self-compassion 74–75; fostering grit 78–79; leisure pastimes 78; meaning-making systems 75–77; self-affirmation 73–74; self-narrative 72–73; sharing learning 79
intentional enrichment 22–23
isomorphism 50, 51–52

jasmine 28
job satisfaction 107
Jung, C. 52, 91

Kahneman, D. 83
Kaminsky, P. 32
Kellogg, J. 52
Kim, J. 44
kinesthetic/sensory level 18
Kohn, M. 41
Kondo, M. 51

label-locked thinking 72
left-brain cognitive process 71
Lehrer, Jonah 100
LEM *see* life enrichment model (LEM)
Life-Changing Magic of Tidying Up, The 51
life-enhancing practices 65
life enrichment model: movement 39

life enrichment model (LEM) 2, 3, 17; benefits 11–14; circle assessment 23; creativity 95; creativity 21–22; dynamic balance 24; emotion 20–21, 61; enriched life practice 105; intellect 21; intentional enrichment 22–23; optimal health path way to 18; pattern and routine 49–48; self-actualizing tendency 21; sensation 27; sensation 18–20; structure of the 18; through intellect 71; through symbolism 83
Lifestyle Medicine Institute 78
limbic system or the mammalian brain 20
listening to music 34
low-arousal colors 29
low/high-arousal colors 29
Luthans, F. 106

Malinowski, A. J. 4
Mandala coloring 52
massage 31
Mata, J. 42
meaning-making systems 75–77
meditation 46
Merton, T. 50
micro-self-care practices 7
Montessori, M. 27
music 34, 49
myths 89–90

narrative network 35
Necessity of Art, The 85
Neff, K. 74
negative mood 52

Oates, J.C. 50
olfactory sensation 28
optical illusions 55
optimal health: definition 14–15; path way to 18
optimism 107
oxytocin 31

peace lily (plant) 30
physical activity/movement: antidepressant effects 41; art experience through 41; and art reflections 47; benefits of exercise 40; and brain 44, 45; and cognitive functioning 42; dance 45–46; enhanced sleep 42; fatigue 43–44; positive benefits 42; and positive emotions 41; rhythmic movement 44–45; strength 43; yoga 41
physical fatigue 5
physiological arousal 29
play 97–98; types of 97
poetry 90–91
Poetry Foundation 91
positive emotion 27, 62, 63–64, 98, 108
Post Traumatic Growth (PTG) 6
Post Traumatic Stress Disorder (PTSD) 4
Power of Myth, The 89
problem solving 71
problem-solving strategies 14
professional burnout 4, 72
pro-inflammatory proteins 108
psychological capital 107
psychological immune system 73
psychologically therapeutic effect 17
psychologist 2
PTG *see* Post Traumatic Growth (PTG)
PTSD *see* Post Traumatic Stress Disorder (PTSD)

Rat Park, art reflection 16
replenishing the well 107–108
representational diversity 54–56
reptilian brain 18
resilience 107
respire 15
right-hemisphere process 83
rituals 87; family 88–89; social and religious 88
routines and patterns, LEM: and art reflection 58–59; art therapy 54; and behavior 51; circle aid meditation 52; comfort of 50–51; doodling 54; isomorphism 51–52; lines aid meditation 51–54; Mandala coloring 52; representational diversity 55;

setting boundaries 57–58; sharing and perception 54–56
Ruud, E. 68

satisfaction 27
secondary traumatic stress 4; prevention and treatment of 6–7
self-actualizing tendency 21
self-affirmation 73–74
self-care: practices 21
self-compassion 74–75; elements of 75
self-confidence 41
self-control miracle 40
self-referential thought 86
self-reflection 68
self-reflective activity 58
self-stigma 72
Seligman, M. P. 62, 63
sensation 18–20; auditory sensation and silence 33–34; and the brain 35; olfactory 28; sensual pleasure 35–37; sharing aroma 29; sharing beauty 30–31; sharing music 34; sharing touch 31; tactile 31; taste 32–33; visual 29–30
sensory actions and art reflections 38
sensual experience 27
sensual pleasure 35–37
sleep 42
sliver queen (plant) 30
social media 30
spirituality 15
stress 41, 52
stress ball 44–45
stress inoculation 42, 46
stressors 42
stress syndromes 8
symbolic thinking 83
symbolism: and art reflection 93; dreams 91; family rituals 88–89; illustrated books 90; myths 89–90; poetry 90–91; sharing symbols 87; social and religious rituals 88; synchronicity 91–92
symbolism: intellect and 21

tactile sensation 31
taste sensation 32–33
Taylor, Barbara Brown 37
tense energy 43
trauma 72

U-shaped model 42

vicarious resilience 68
vicarious traumatization 4
virtuous cycle 12
visual sensation 29–30

walk 42, 43
wavelength spectrum 29
wide margins 109–110
Widow's Story, A 50
work–life balance 76
workouts 41

yoga 41
Youssef-Morgan, C. M. 106

Zentangle™ 52–54